# THE DOULA GUIDE TO BIRTH

# THE DOULA GUIDE TO BIRTH

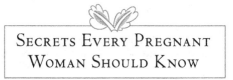

SECRETS EVERY PREGNANT
WOMAN SHOULD KNOW

Ananda Lowe
and
Rachel Zimmerman

BANTAM BOOKS

This book contains general information, ideas, and techniques that have been successfully used by many families to enhance their birth experiences. Please check with your own health-care provider(s) and use your own good judgment in order to determine what information applies to your specific situation and which ideas and techniques are appropriate for you. Every situation is different. We make no guarantees or assurance of any kind to anyone. Only you can make the important decisions you will face during pregnancy, labor, and birth. The information in this book is presented in the hope that it will inspire you to seek the best and safest options for you, your baby, and your family.

A Bantam Books Trade Paperback Original

Copyright © 2009 by Ananda Lowe and Rachel Zimmerman

Published in the United States by Bantam Books, an imprint of The Random House Publishing Group, a division of Random House, Inc., New York.

BANTAM BOOKS and the rooster colophon are registered trademarks of Random House, Inc.

Library of Congress Cataloging-in-Publication Data

Lowe, Ananda, 1969–
The doula guide to birth : secrets every pregnant woman should know / Ananda Lowe and Rachel Zimmerman.
p. cm.
Includes bibliographical references and index.
ISBN 978-0-553-38526-7 (pbk.) — ISBN 978-0-553-90659-2 (ebook)
1. Doulas.    2. Childbirth.    I. Zimmerman, Rachel, 1964–    II. Title.
RG950.L688 2009
618.4—dc22                                    2009001764

www.bantamdell.com

Book design by Catherine Leonardo

146122990

To my mother, Rochelle Lowe, with love;
and for Ilana Stein, a doula ancestor now

—AL

To my daughters,
Sophia and Julia, the bright stars in my life;
and to my mother, Selma Rabow Zimmerman—now I know

—RZ

# ⟬ TABLE OF CONTENTS ⟬

# INTRODUCTION

## *Ananda*

I am an experienced doula (pronounced *doo*-luh), or professional labor assistant, which means my life is immersed in the world of birth.

I've given intensive support to women and couples in labor in their homes and at nearly every hospital and birth center in the greater Boston area, where I live.

I have helped many mothers figure out when their labors were "real," saving them hours of waiting at the hospital at the wrong time. I've guided them to sleep when their labors went on for days, so they could have the stamina to finish the job.

I've supported women as they delivered their babies on their hands and knees, in a tub of water, flat on their backs, standing up, on operating tables, and in a car.

I have sat with women as they revealed their family secrets, and as they wept with the frustration or joy of becoming mothers themselves.

I've given hours of massage, in place of pain medications, to laboring moms. I have gently closed their hospital room doors (which are normally left wide open) hundreds and hundreds of times—this preserves the calm in their rooms, and keeps the commotion of a busy labor and delivery floor outside.

One-on-one with a mother, a doula becomes an extension of the birthing woman's intuition. The doula senses what her client needs moment by moment, in a way no other healthcare provider, divided among multiple patients in labor, can.

I have also been a certified lactation counselor, a licensed massage therapist specializing in pregnancy, and a postpartum doula, a helper at home in the newborn period—which is how I met my cowriter, Rachel. I worked with Rachel when her second daughter was an infant, and while we were bonding in that role, we decided we should share our wisdom with a larger audience.

There now are thousands of doulas all over the United States and the world. I have talked with many of them throughout my years in this profession. Most choose this career after having a wonderful or challenging experience giving birth themselves. They are excited to pass along what they learned in birth to other mothers. And there are those, like me, who feel pulled to begin this fascinating work while we're still childless.

Some become doulas because we are young and curious feminists, eager to learn about women's bodies and rights. Some of us have "always known" we want to give birth eventually, while others may have bypassed the traditional path of young wife and mom.

It feels thrilling as well as poignant to become a doula before giving birth. I am lucky, because in my mid-thirties, I am one of the only members of my group of friends to have had the chance to be present at someone else's birth. It has been amazing for me too, watching dozens of mothers figure out how to go through labor without ever having seen it themselves.

In other places and times in history, this would be different. All women would be like doulas and have the chance to witness births, starting as young girls. This would help plenty when it came time for them to give birth, too.

As doulas, there is yet another reason we may be drawn to this work—which is, of course, that all of us have a mother. And even though for some of us, our relationships with our mothers might have been difficult in some way (or perhaps because of that fact), we love our job, supporting families in their raw and awesome newness.

As for me, I was the young and curious feminist, not the girl who'd "always known" motherhood would be for me (it is possible to be both, of course). I needed a new job because my work, in the stressful worlds of advertising photography and waitressing, was not something I could stick with for the long haul.

An idealist, I looked for a job that would somehow let me use my experience organizing projects to help people in a deeper way in their lives. ALACE, the doula organization, posted an ad in the local women's newspaper looking for help, and I was hired. I didn't know a thing about birth at twenty-five, but I loved soaking up the information from day one.

When I was hired, but before my job even started, I im-mediately began quizzing friends and acquaintances: What position did you give birth in? Did you have a midwife? I wasn't exactly sure what a midwife was, and I'd never heard of a doula before. But something was sparked in me to learn all about the fascinating options women can have (and that we've often sadly been in the dark about, or denied).

I began organizing doula trainings around the country, by phone, from a teensy home office shared with my two cowork-ers. We hired experienced labor assistants to teach the train-ings. I attended the training seminar myself, after a few months on the job. I remember walking home from the course, a long weekend crammed with explicit birth videos and a couple dozen women in a small room, talking intensely about their bodies, births, and lives.

As I walked home at dusk, and saw my neighbor's preschool-age children running up and down my street, I could only think in amazement, "You were born! And you were born, too!"

We had introduced ourselves at the workshop, and I said, "My name is Ananda, and I'm taking this class because birth is about healing." It was a vague and innocent statement, but somehow I knew it was deeply true for me.

Later that year, a good friend invited me to attend her birth, my first experience doing so. When the day came I supported her eagerly, after getting over my initial panic when I received the call at dawn to come to the hospital. The second time, another friend was having her hair done by her eight-months-pregnant stylist, and she volunteered me to be the woman's doula. Through word of mouth, I began getting more and more requests to attend labors professionally.

———————

Turning into a doula is a bit like being pregnant—it takes months to start to absorb what you're really getting yourself into.

It was mind-boggling how much there was to learn: how insurance pressures and medical fads (not science) often control choices doctors and families make; how little I knew about other options, like giving birth at home; that there's as much to know about baby-feeding as there is about birth; and so much more. After more than thirteen intense years I'm still learning, and still not bored.

In my early doula days, I felt tongue-tied when people asked, "How did you get into this, why do you do this work?" Sometimes I talked about my experience of advocating for my own health care in my twenties, which taught me the vital importance of having someone as a guide, if possible. Sometimes I tried to describe what I'd discovered about being present with a woman on the day in her life when she is most powerful.

I thought maybe I should give a simple answer about what a miracle it is to be there when a new life enters the world. That didn't really capture all that it meant to me, but seemed to be the easiest way to reply, or what I assumed people wanted to hear.

Those reasons are true, and part of the answer. But it's only in the last year or so that another important piece of the puzzle has become obvious to me.

My mother gave birth alone in the 1960s, as did many of the moms of my peers, without her own mother or the fathers of her babies allowed to be present. (My mother was married twice.)

She'd heard of Lamaze breathing, and she tried to invent it on the spot, by herself in labor. She figured breastfeeding was a good idea, so she taught herself how, also alone, by reading a book she checked out of a Los Angeles public library while pregnant with my oldest sister in 1963. Cloth diapers were all that existed, and she went to the Laundromat every other day to wash dozens of them herself.

Mom went back to work several weeks after giving birth, not because she was superwoman, but because her office-manager job was a more stable source of income than her husbands' work. These were hard marriages, and a supportive friend or relative nearby would have been a great boon, but it didn't happen that way.

I realize now how much it means to me personally to help families have support as they welcome a child. And in the twenty-first century, women are still mostly left alone in birth, albeit now with their husbands and loved ones—who deserve and need support as much as laboring moms.

What a difference it makes to simply have someone who is fully there for you on the day your world transforms. I describe this to my clients as "the way everyone used to always give birth," with a devoted female labor companion. (In the long line of history, only since about the 1930s have mothers been separated from their support networks, when birth was moved from the home to the hospital.) In some cultures it was an all-women event, and in others dads were normally present at birth. Either way, the neighbor women came right over, to firmly guard and humbly assist the way.

Doulas want to bring this tradition back—because it is human nature, because it is less scary and lonely, because labor is shorter and less painful, because doulas help strengthen new families, because we were not designed to be left alone in birth. Because the gift of total love and care is what allows us to say, like I did as a naïve young doula, "Birth is about healing."

———

Studies show that what happens during birth may shape women's feelings about themselves as mothers for years to come. Having a baby takes all of one's strength, and women have described the achievement of giving birth as empowering.

On the other hand, when birth is difficult or disappointing, women sometimes wonder whether they are at fault, and "different" from other mothers. When women go through labor with a doula, they report feeling more positively about their births and having a better ability to take care of their babies. All mothers deserve to feel this way.

I often tell my clients: "There is just one society of mothers. And every mother is part of it, regardless of how she birthed." This is not to erase the experience of a woman who, for example, gave birth by cesarean when she expected to have a smoother labor. (I tell these moms that far from having inferior births, they deserve to be admired. Usually they labored devotedly, in tougher situations than average, *and* had surgery on top of it.)

My most recent experience at a cesarean was with a caring, veteran obstetrician. She has been working since around the year of my birth, when one in twenty babies was delivered by surgery, until today, when that number has soared to almost one in three.

She explained, "I know as doctors, we are performing too many cesareans now. In some cases, it's a necessary operation. The trouble is, at this point in medicine, we're unable to be sure which operations are the necessary ones."

How did this get lost, the knowledge of what mothers and babies need, in the space of one generation?

For moms, an unplanned cesarean is sometimes more challenging emotionally than a vaginal birth, and at times these women describe feeling left out among their friends. Whether they are my clients, my friends, or strangers whom I meet, I find myself reminding these women they too are full members of the society of mothers.

I'd like to mention the treasured midwife Ina May Gaskin, who has made legends out of women's birth stories. First she did this in her classic book *Spiritual Midwifery,* and more recently in the book *Ina May's Guide to Childbirth.*

In Gaskin's books, mothers often give birth in seeming ecstasy. I've heard some readers say they felt let down because their own births couldn't measure up to the happy tales in these books. But on looking closer, you can see there is certainly hardship in some of Ina May's stories. Some babies are born too ill to survive, or labor goes on almost unthinkably long.

The difference about those births is that they mostly take place at the famous alternative birth center Mrs. Gaskin founded in Tennessee. It's not that their physical labors are somehow magically easier. These women seem to be on equal footing, as strong mother-goddesses, and it's because of the birth center's brilliant philosophy of support, not because these are all perfect birth scenarios.

In the same way, I believe *all* mothers are part of one sisterhood and deserve to feel proud of their births. This is whether they give birth with or without a doula, with or without surgery, with or without drugs, with or without knowledge of their bodies and options, with or without husbands or partners, with or without live and healthy babies, with or without hospitals and doctors, with or without even being awake—and with or without any support at all.

All mothers belong, and the stories of their births matter deeply. The day on which a baby is born (and therefore a mother is born, and a family is born), is a day that will be remembered forever. Decades after my mother gave birth, she remembers the exact words her nurses said to her and their tone of voice during those hours. And she always tells me she loved how I stared at her right after I was born.

So many other things matter about being a mother, surely, beyond the day of giving birth. But birth is never a small event. It is the event that changes your life permanently, from that moment forward. It's the event that demands your attention, mentally, emotionally, and physically, in a way that nothing else can in life. And the way birth is handled can affect women and their families long into the future.

I once made a remark to Jessica Porter, the former director of ALACE. Jessica's babies were young, and I shared something I often tell my pregnant clients about labor: "It's probably the hardest thing you'll ever do, and I want you to know you can do it." Jessica chuckled and replied, "Well, labor is the hardest thing you'll ever do in life—up until that day," referring to the demands of new parenthood. Indeed.

Birth matters. It brings us into being, on many levels. Many mothers report they often look back to the day they gave birth and say, "Well, if I got through birth, I can get through whatever trying experience is happening today."

For myself, as a doula, I have a phrase that echoes in my own head when I am facing a challenge in life. Many times I've said to myself, "I have the courage inside me that women have during birth." Though I don't yet know whether I'll physically give birth in life, *knowing* I have this strength is an automatic part of me now. It is the same courage that is needed to make it through deep loss, personal change, and the pursuit of our greatest dreams in life.

All women have this strength. (All men do too, because they are human, and because, as the poets William Shakespeare and Adrienne Rich said, they too are "of woman born.")

Perhaps that strength is what really makes us mothers—whether we are newly pregnant, raising a houseful of kids, united with or separated from our babies, or even childless (what I call mothers-in-spirit). The society of mothers is one larger family, so to speak. Welcome to this family.

———

Doulas exist as guardians for families while they're being born. As you'll see in the pages ahead, births with labor assistants result in healthier babies and moms, fewer surgeries and drugs in labor, less postpartum depression, and stronger marital and family bonds. Research and science show us that. And we know it from our own experience.

In fact, many doulas love the saying, "Peace on earth begins at birth." Birth is perhaps the most important event of our lives—and not just because it is when a new person enters the world, but because it is the start of our families and our first profound relationships.

I'm delighted to have grown up as a woman, inside the doula movement, during the years the doula movement has been growing up itself. I'm happy that my mother has enjoyed hearing about my work so much, and my father did too while he was living.

During my seven years as assistant director of ALACE, we moved out of the home office to larger quarters, and I organized trainings that enabled thousands of individuals across the United States and Canada to become doulas. It was an honor to be part of creating the doula movement in this way. Women—and a few men—participated in doula trainings from Montana to Manhattan, from San Diego to South Carolina, and from Toronto to Texas. They went on to support the births of mothers in all circumstances, from celebrities and doctors to homeless and incarcerated women, ranging in age from their teens to their fifties.

To our readers, I still want to say what I have said for many years: *you can do it*. You can accomplish the amazing event of birth in joy, you can pursue and even achieve your greatest dreams, and I hope you'll be able to do so with the full support that you—and your marvelous families—most truly deserve.

## *Rachel*

By the time I was ready to give birth to my second daughter at age forty-one, I thought I was a pro. I didn't think I needed a refresher birthing class, where we had (laughably) held ice cubes to simulate the pain of childbirth. I had no use for yet another prenatal advice book telling me I'd gained too much or too little weight. I knew enough by now about birthing balls and water births and breathing. After all, I'd already given birth to a healthy child and raised her for nearly three years, through twenty-four months of breastfeeding, two months traipsing through Tuscany, many nights slithering out of her room on my belly so the creaky floor wouldn't wake her, and extended potty training. (OK, she turned three and still preferred to poop in a diaper.)

So when my water broke that second time, on a Monday evening, I was clearheaded and thought I knew what was ahead. With my wise-woman savvy, I coolly packed a much different bag than I had the first time around. Instead of a pretty nightie, I grabbed one of my husband's soft, extralarge

T-shirts (better for absorbing blood); rather than a novel, I brought the cell phone charger (nobody obeys the hospital ban). And I packed the book of baby names since we were still arguing, with no common ground, about what to call her. (We chose our first child's name, Sophia Mariel, gleefully and easily on the beach in St. John Island.)

Of course, there would be similarities in the two births. I was lucky to have both of my children delivered by an amazing obstetrician, Beth Hardiman, one of the last solo practitioners left in Cambridge, Massachusetts, and as far as I'm concerned, a medical goddess and also a strong proponent of doulas. Ultracompetent as a doctor, but with a therapist's patience and a masseuse's magic touch, Dr. Hardiman was right there with me both times, dousing me with olive oil so I wouldn't need an episiotomy and handling every question, every scream, every doubt with grace and the skill of a top surgeon.

In truth, though, the two births felt completely different—twenty-four hours of labor the first time, seven hours the second; an epidural for Sophia's birth, none for Julia's. But the thing that connected both events was this: each time I had to confront the unexpected amidst the most physically and emotionally charged situation imaginable.

That's where the doulas came in. Before, during, and after both births I had professional women around who helped me in ways I couldn't have imagined. Jane Look, my first doula, had already worked with my two close friends, Amy and Sally, and was always available when I was pregnant: she helped me work out a birth plan, gave me advice on how to sleep despite my physical discomfort, and offered exercises which actually helped turn my upright baby facedown just before her birth.

After my water broke but before active labor, we met our doctor at Mount Auburn Hospital and she told us to go home and relax. Jane agreed. So we went to a dinner party in

Newton, a nearby town, as planned and had a lovely meal of salmon and celeriac soup while I frequented the bathroom to change the towel I'd stuffed between my legs.

The next morning, as the contractions got stronger and more frequent, we checked in to Mount Auburn. Jane was there and we spent hours walking up and down the hospital's back stairs and sitting on the birthing ball; Jane fed me ice chips to fend off the nausea I experienced and on hands and knees we helped alleviate my back labor. No one thing Jane did on its own was particularly miraculous, but she was right there, and quick to offer various ways to ease my pain and comfort me. Unlike everyone else in our immediate circle— my husband, my doctor, my parents, my in-laws—Jane had no agenda except me.

I figured this out when it came to dealing with pain relief. Seth and I had talked a lot about wanting to avoid drugs and give birth to our baby naturally. That's why we took the birthing class, and, in large part, why we hired Jane.

Not everyone agreed with us. My father, for instance, a philosophy professor and avid consumer of pharmaceuticals for every possible discomfort, was mortified that we planned to give birth naturally. "But there are such great drugs for that," he'd said. His voice was in my head when, around nine PM on March 3, after over twenty-one hours of labor and still only dilated about 3 or 4 centimeters, Dr. Hardiman suggested the drug Pitocin to speed things up. In a malleable state, I said yes. But knowing this would intensify contractions that were already pushing me to the edge, I decided I wanted an epidural, even though my written plan was clearly against it. My husband and I had envisioned this moment. But a birth plan on paper is nothing compared to a birth, live. My husband, Seth, an engineer, tried to stick to the plan a little longer. He gently urged me to hold out. "You can do it." I began to wonder about my own ability to make the right call at this point and I resented the pressure to be a superstar. I kept thinking, *I've hit a wall and I am too exhausted to deal with more pain.*

Our doula, Jane, sensed that my indecision was fueling my anxiety, making the pain even worse. Quietly, she said, "It's OK to get the epidural if you feel you need it. It will help the pain." I held out for one more major contraction and then realized I wanted help. I got the epidural, slept three hours with my husband by my side and Jane on the floor, woke up dilated nearly 10 centimeters, pushed with no pain but still feeling the baby move down the birth canal, and twenty minutes later gave birth to my gorgeous child Sophia.

I didn't bother with a birth plan the second time around. And I debated whether to hire a doula at all since I felt like I knew what was coming. Jane had gotten quite ill and was no longer working. She recommended Joyce Kimball, whom I decided to hire, and who spent hours talking with me on the phone and by e-mail about how to prevent the intense nausea I'd felt during my first labor, how to prepare myself better for postpartum depression, and how to talk to Sophia about the new baby.

Still, the second time around had a whole different feel. The giddy, "miracle of birth" aura had dissipated; I just wanted to be done with it and go home with Sophia and her new sister. One of the first things I said to Dr. Hardiman when I arrived at Mount Auburn Hospital was: "Tell me when it's too late for the epidural." It had been so effective for me last time, with no negative side effects, I thought I'd probably end up using it again.

But nature intervened.

My second labor was typical in that it was much faster. I got to the hospital around nine PM and spent the first hour or two chatting with the nurses about baby names, polling them to see if "Katrina" was an acceptable choice in the fall of 2005. (They thought it wasn't.) A couple of hours later I was in the tub, moaning away. Joyce massaged my lower back and covered me with the soft shirt when I got a bad case of the chills. She was there with me when Seth ran out to check on Sophia, asleep in an empty breastfeeding room with my brother-in-law at the other end of the hospital. A videotape taken around eleven-thirty PM shows me on the birthing ball grimacing up to the camera: "Honey, I don't know how much more of the pain I can take. It hurts."

After only three hours of active labor, I was about 6 centimeters dilated and Dr. Hardiman thought an epidural might take too long so she suggested an injection of fentanyl, a painkiller. They gave me a low dose, which did nothing. When, at one AM, I finally told Dr. Hardiman I wanted the epidural, she said, "Too late." In the fetal position on my side, after about four more contractions that convinced me this was the last child I'd be having, I pushed against a fierce burning that I was numb to the first time around. Joyce helped me stop hyperventilating, continued to massage me between contractions, and let me grab on to her as I screamed, and then screamed louder. Forty minutes later, around one-fifty AM, Julia was born, essentially drug-free. Some women report they've had orgasms during childbirth; that would have been nice. But for me, it was more like the biggest bowel movement on earth, and very satisfying in its own way. Afterward, I felt like a total jock.

Joyce and I had talked a lot about how I could avoid falling into depression as I had after Sophia was born. When my first daughter was young, Seth and I had a rough time, often getting tangled up in the kind of sleep-deprived fights about child-rearing at three AM that can unravel a marriage.

One thing Joyce recommended was a postpartum doula, someone who could help us as needed in those first wild weeks. I don't think it's exaggerating to say Ananda, an experienced birth and postpartum doula, helped keep my marriage and my life intact. I felt guilty and indulgent when I first talked to her about doing some cooking, straightening up around the house, and watching the baby so I could get back to exercising and hang out with Sophia. And deep down, I never stopped feeling that I really should be doing it all myself. My divorced mother did it; my mother-in-law did it. Even women who can pay for this kind of help feel like they have to do it on their own. But then I think how lucky I am that I've tapped into this world of women supporting women, all of us passing along advice to one another about how we can focus on loving and nurturing our kids, improving our relationships with our spouses, and doing meaningful work while also taking care of ourselves. Leaving the laundry to someone else once in a while isn't a crime, I kept repeating.

With Ananda in my house, rather than postpartum insanity, I experienced something akin to postpartum elation. I actually had moments—rare for me, a dark, cynical New Yorker—when I thought, *I have it all: two healthy daughters, a job at a great newspaper, a wonderful husband—and a clean house.*

Indeed, I've come to think that the birth of a child is a lot like a wedding. We're racked with anxiety over the event itself—will the dress fit? Will the divorced parents kill each other? Will it rain? We get so fixated on and whipped up over the big day, trying to match it against the elaborate fantasy, that we don't give enough thought to what comes on day two. Of course, birth is important—it's the beginning of family. And weddings are important too; they set the tone for a life together. But what comes later is even bigger, and potentially darker: the realization that marriage and parenting can be terribly difficult, with little resemblance to the dream.

Between the sleep deprivation, the loss of romance and freedom, the inability to soothe every cry, and the complete cluelessness of new parents, I sometimes wonder how it is women continue to have children. But the next moment I think about having a third.

One night after many in which Sophia simply wouldn't sleep, I threw myself onto the floor, literally crumpled into a heap, saying I couldn't do it anymore. All that accomplished was to frighten my husband and create a moment that required much discussion in subsequent therapy sessions.

I didn't want to repeat that scene with my second child. Ananda was no magician: but caring for the baby while I did yoga, cooking a few healthy meals each week, taking out the garbage, and tidying up the house, she gave me space to be a good mother. And between chores, she counseled me on engorged breasts, hemorrhoids, frustratingly slow weight loss, and the crazy cycles of annoyance and gratitude I felt toward my husband. She was a true lifeline as our family grew.

I started writing this introduction while nursing three-month-old Julia in bed on a chilly March afternoon as three-year-old Sophia napped. I hadn't yet showered. Only a few years earlier, as a single, ambitious reporter at the *Wall Street Journal,* my life had been consumed with planning a trip to Africa to report a story, figuring out which shuttle flight I could make to visit my boyfriend (now husband), and wondering if I could get a spot in the seven PM aerobics class. In motherhood, a single day can go by with no perceptible accomplishments, except that I've managed to change the blowout-poop diaper and sweep most of the brown rice off the floor. But those endless days can also bring profound tenderness. "Sophia is a star," I wrote in my diary four days after her birth. "She's gorgeous, wise, knowing, and when she sleeps in my bed at night, my love is so deep and complete, I feel there is no food, no air, no water more sustaining." Seth, trying to soothe the baby in those first days, relied on his guy instincts and walked her around the house whispering all the rules of his favorite sport, Ultimate Frisbee—a true act of love.

My friend Sally, who found our first birth doula, Jane, and e-mailed her every day during pregnancy, says she couldn't have sustained her thirty-six-hour, drug-free labor without Jane's help. When Sally brought over a luscious chicken potpie after Sophia's birth, she described the awesome sweetness of new motherhood: "You thought you knew what love was, well, now you know."

And when I see Julia gaze starstruck at her big sister dancing, with a look that is part awe and part wonder, I know there is even more love in the house with these two girls.

I try to control a great deal about my children's lives, but I know I can't care for them alone. With compassion, patience, and calm, doulas can help us remember to trust what we already know instinctively, and help us learn to be flexible when faced with the unknown. With this support, we can love our children and our families more deeply. In the end, there is no perfect birth, just like there is no perfect marriage or perfect child. Doulas are not about achieving perfection; they are more about clearing a path that will bring you home.

# THE DOULA GUIDE TO BIRTH

I

# DOULAS ARE GREAT PAIN RELIEF

*I did not end up taking pain medicine in labor, but I almost feel like I did. Instead, my partner and my doula took turns massaging me for my whole labor, which lasted three days. While I was pregnant, our doula taught us some easy ways to use touch, and she said our homework was to practice cuddling, which was fine with us!*

*By the time labor came, my partner and I knew how to keep touching naturally, and it turned out to be a great relief for the pain. My labor was a lot of work, but our doula was there every moment, and the nurturing from her and my partner really was like a wonderful drug in itself.*

—Sylvia, 29, real-estate agent, mother of two

Giving birth with a doula is the most important trend of modern maternity care. The word comes from the Greek, translated to mean "slave" or "servant." It was first used in the 1970s by the anthropologist Dana Raphael, who adopted it to mean a helper of new mothers. (Though some Greeks and doulas are not crazy about the word, it has become commonplace.)

Doulas are today's new experts in labor. Trained as professional birth companions, they act as highly skilled guides through the dramatic forces of labor. Using a combination of wit, science, and the ancient (but nearly lost) art of human support in birth, doulas have a powerful effect on the first major rite of passage we all must complete: being born.

And we like to think of it this way too: *doulas can be your best form of pain relief in birth.*

Their philosophy is to stay with you constantly, from start to finish in active labor, without taking breaks or changing shifts (which is not possible for most doctors, nurses, or midwives in hospitals). They come equipped with the ability to remain calm as the waves of labor intensify, to provide solid guidance for new dads and loved ones, to advocate for you with skill, and to remember all of the available labor techniques, with clear insight about when it's wise to use each one.

Birth doulas, also known as labor assistants, may guide you in: breathing methods or relaxation images, intensive emotional coaching, feedback on whether your labor pain is within normal range, and ways to actually sleep during the marathon work of labor. They may offer techniques to prevent the extra pain of back labor; delivery positions that use gravity in your favor; and even advanced specialties, such as hypnotherapy for pain relief, professional massage therapy, or acupuncture.

Doulas can help first-time parents give birth with less fear, help experienced mothers find new strength, and help women giving birth after a cesarean have more options.

In 2002 and 2006, the respected organization Childbirth Connection issued two groundbreaking reports, *Listening to Mothers I* and *II,* the first-ever surveys of women's own experiences giving birth across the United States. And when it came to labor support, mothers rated a doula's help more effective than that of any other health-care provider.

In most cases, a doula works independently—directly for

you—which allows her to openly serve as your advocate. Also, doulas are often the only maternity-care providers who have worked at every hospital in town. This gives them a rare bird's-eye view of important birthing trends, advances, and setbacks in your community.

Doulas have something new to say about birth. Amid climbing cesarean rates and other national and worldwide debates in maternal health care, the doula movement has been taking hold as a way for pregnant women to regain more control over their birthing process.

If you've already decided to use a doula, this book will help you make the most of what she has to offer. If you are new to this revolutionary trend, we'll be providing information that will help you decide whether to work with a doula. And even if you are not able to work with one, you will benefit from the doula wisdom that can help you have a more empowered birth.

In writing this book, we stand on the shoulders of other authors who first introduced the world to the idea of doulas, including Dr. John Kennell, Dr. Marshall Klaus, and Phyllis Klaus, CSW, the pioneering researchers who have studied and written about the benefits of doulas for the past three decades. The Klauses and Dr. Kennell collected much of the data on doulas that is accepted in the field now. Multiple studies show that the presence of a labor assistant *can cut your chances in half* for encountering many problems and interventions in birth. Most impressive, this includes the need for such common but major medical procedures as epidurals and cesareans.

Our goal is to build on this work and share with the public the actual techniques, skills, and trade secrets that allow doulas to achieve such remarkable results. As doulas shape their emerging profession, they are contributing original ideas to central issues such as how long labor should take, the most effective ways to prepare for normal and unusual levels of pain in labor, and much more.

*The Doula Guide to Birth* is a book for all pregnant women—single, married, partnered, heterosexual, lesbian, and mothers whose baby will be adopted by another family. Doulas benefit all types of families by honoring their choices, relieving them of the pressure of having to be labor experts, and allowing them to give birth with the security of a familiar guide. Also, partners, fathers, and loved ones are invited to read all sections of this book, and chapter 2 speaks directly to them.

While the authors of this book live in the United States, where the modern doula movement was born, the doula trend has become an international phenomenon. That is why you will see references to birthing customs in various countries, meant to address our readers globally, and to remind us all of our connection to mothers around the world.

## SUPPORT IS WHAT GETS WOMEN THROUGH LABOR

For ages, mothers gave birth surrounded by women who knew them well, whether it was a couple of local wise women or a crowd of female relatives and neighbors. When birth was moved into hospitals in the last century, this took a heavy toll on women's ability to rely on a personal support system in labor. Medical doctors did not realize that isolating women made birth more difficult and painful.

Birth is normally the most profound event of our lives. Like running a marathon yet even more intense, it is easier to accomplish with the steady faith of admirers and friends, and the know-how of those who have been there before. While modern maternity care often leaves mothers and fathers alone in labor, doulas focus their attention on you every moment of the way. This kind of social support provides a sense of security that may be the most important factor for getting through birth.

The doula approach is usually not to leave your delivery room unless it's requested, or she needs a bathroom break or a meal. At those moments, she gives her reassurances that she will quickly return. Mothers in labor are often keenly aware of when their supporters are missing from the room. Depending on the style of a particular doula, as well as your own needs and preferences, a doula may offer support by being a calm and quiet presence during many hours of labor, or she might gently coach and talk you through nearly every contraction.

Human support relieves pain, reduces fear of the unknown, and makes labor manageable in a way that isn't possible when that support is removed. In fact, throughout most of history, human support was entirely what women relied on to ease the way through childbearing (pain drugs simply were not available). And the tradition of women helping women benefited more than the laboring mother. It also benefited her supporters; other women learned what to expect when they would give birth, and they also gained confidence in their ability to help someone through labor—an important achievement in itself.

In recent decades, ordinary women saw the need for doulas and began answering the call. They looked to trailblazers like Rahima Baldwin Dancy of Informed Homebirth/Informed Birth & Parenting (later to become ALACE), Paulina Perez, and Penny Simkin of Doulas of North America (later to become DONA International), who were among the first to begin teaching women how to support laboring mothers. Doulas are usually trained by attending an intensive seminar over several days and then studying textbooks on birth. Ultimately though, a doula's knowledge comes from an experience most doctors and nurses never get to have—staying with women nonstop through their entire labors. The rise of doulas is a powerful example of women taking grassroots action to help themselves and other women.

## DOULAS: THE BEST MEDICINE

Although doulas are not trained in medical schools, they have an important effect on birth, medically.

Some women seek a labor assistant to help them achieve a goal of natural childbirth. However, even if that is not a mother's main goal, a doula has the effect of reducing the likelihood of medical interventions, along with their possible risks.

According to the Cochrane Collaboration, the respected organization that reviews international clinical research, studies of more than one thousand mothers show that the presence of a doula results in lower rates of all types of pain medicine, cesareans, and deliveries with forceps or vacuums. Smaller studies show that rates of other procedures are reduced with a doula, including breaking the bag of waters artificially and the use of drugs to speed labor. (These were controlled studies comparing groups of women who were otherwise similar.)

In countries including the United States and Canada, the most common form of pain relief in birth has become the epidural, a type of anesthesia that numbs the body from the waist down. But increasingly, women are learning they can also have the support of a doula, instead of or in addition to medication, and they're reporting more positive birth experiences—including less pain. All women wonder how they will manage labor pain; a doula helps settle their fears. And while anesthesia and surgery have become common in labor, medical procedures for birth (like those for any health condition) have potential side effects.

The *Listening to Mothers* surveys showed that after giving birth, the majority of women nationally said they had not understood the risks of the medical interventions they received in labor. As numerous doulas have observed, when doctors discuss consent for an epidural with pregnant women, they do not always fully explain one of its most important side effects:

*epidurals lower the blood pressure of one in three mothers, and therefore lower blood flow and oxygen to the baby.* This can create changes in the baby's heart rate which may be seen as "fetal distress," a cause of further interventions and cesareans.

According to researchers at Harvard Medical School, effects of epidurals can include an increase in problems with pushing the baby out, and more difficulties with newborn health and behavior; this may include more breastfeeding problems, though this is debated among health-care professionals. Some women feel psychological unease due to being less able to move their bodies once they receive an epidural. Epidurals can be valuable—for instance, they may allow women with severe labor pain to relax tense muscles for a smoother labor; and unlike drugs from earlier eras, epidurals permit mothers to remain conscious and awake—but there is reason to reconsider using them automatically.

In some studies, women with doulas report less pain in labor than women without doulas. This is noteworthy not only because it shows the pain-relieving effects of doulas, but because mothers with doulas are more likely to give birth without needing epidurals, yet they still report *less* pain.

A doula guides you in using comfort techniques that are known to decrease pain in labor, including being upright, walking, touch, and the use of warm showers and baths (hydrotherapy). We think of these excellent methods as the "labor techniques any woman can use," without needing any special training in advance.

Childbirth classes may teach these techniques, yet when it comes to the reality and the intensity of actual labor, women and their loved ones may forget or lose confidence in their ability to make use of these methods while alone. Studies show that mothers who use these techniques rate them as some of the most effective pain-relief methods, yet they are tried by the smallest number of women. A doula gives constant reminders throughout labor for using these techniques. With a doula, pain relief is increased because labor techniques are actually put to use rather than forgotten.

If you plan or decide to use pain medicine, a doula still performs her normal comfort measures. Her presence can help delay the timing of when the drug is needed, if that is your wish. In these situations, a doula offers the benefit of helping lower the amount of time you would be exposed to the drugs, thereby lowering the possibility of side effects.

> When I arrived at the hospital around four AM, my doctor informed me I was still in very early labor, and he gave me the option to go home. I was nervous about whether I could handle that on my own, and I wondered if I should just check into the hospital and get an epidural right away.
>
> My doula offered to come home with me if I chose that. We did go home, where my doula massaged me to sleep and I was able to rest for several hours. When I woke up, I could move from room to room, eat, and walk up and down the stairs to help labor along—things I couldn't do at the hospital. With my doula's help, I gained about twelve hours in which I was able to put off the need for an epidural.
>
> —Mikayo, 31, dancer, mother of one

If an epidural is used, a doula can continue providing gentle massage to areas of your body not affected by anesthesia. Massage and other techniques increase relaxation and help lower stress hormones, according to studies by Dr. Tiffany Field of the Touch Research Institute at the University of Miami School of Medicine. During birth, massage can help prevent stress levels from slowing down the labor hormones that are still needed to finish the job.

Some studies show the use of a doula also results in lower

use of the drug Pitocin (known as Syntocinon in some countries), a synthetic version of labor hormones widely used by doctors and midwives to artificially speed up labor. Pitocin creates contractions that can be more painful than natural labor. Therefore, a doula provides pain relief by lowering the chances of Pitocin being used. Current estimates of the use of Pitocin are as high as 50 to 60 percent of births in the United States, and over 20 percent in Britain. With a doula, the use of Pitocin has been shown to be reduced by 40 percent.

According to research conducted by Dr. Kennell and the Klauses, the use of a doula results in labors that are 25 percent shorter. In fact, in their studies, women with doulas had shorter labors than women who received Pitocin or other interventions to hasten labor. Thus, with a doula, pain is reduced because there are significantly fewer hours in which to experience pain.

With a doula, a woman has access to a wider range of techniques to handle the common hurdles of birth, such as being sleep deprived after hours or days of labor, or having a baby who is not lined up in an ideal way in the mother's pelvis. If drugs or medical procedures are needed, a mother can feel more assured that the procedures are likely to be necessary, rather than being used routinely on her.

## DOULAS AND PREMATURITY

Most of the research studies involving doulas have focused on whether labor support leads to decreased interventions, like C-sections and epidurals. But an emerging topic of research is the doula's potential impact on preventing low-birth-weight babies and premature babies born before thirty-seven weeks of gestation.

Prematurity is the leading cause of infant

## ᗧ DOULAS AND PREMATURITY ᗧ

*(continued from previous page)*

mortality in the first month of life, according to the March of Dimes, a nonprofit organization. Children born preterm are also at greater risk of developing serious and long-term illness and developmental delays. Preventing premature birth is a top public health goal.

Can doulas play a role?

A 2003 evaluation of the first four years of the community-based doula pilot project in Chicago—which pairs low-income, at-risk teenage mothers with doulas who support them prenatally, during birth, and postpartum—found that the doula-supported mothers were less likely to have a premature or low-birth-weight baby compared to a matched cohort of mothers across the state. (They were also less likely to have inadequate prenatal care.) Fewer than 5 percent of the babies in the doula project were born prematurely; during the same time period, the average prematurity rate in Illinois was more than 12 percent for all births and significantly higher for teens as well as African-Americans, who represented more than one-third of the participants.

Doula-supported mothers in the Chicago project also reported higher breastfeeding rates, more positive interaction between mothers and newborns, and a greater delay before subsequent pregnancies.

Data from other sites modeled after the Chicago doula project are beginning to confirm these initial findings. For example, research from the data project at the Georgia Campaign for

Adolescent Pregnancy Prevention, or G-CAPP, also found lower rates of premature and low-birth-weight babies. Among 104 teen mothers in the program, age fifteen to nineteen, only five girls, fewer than 5 percent, had preterm babies. In Georgia in 2006, the premature birth rate for girls fifteen to seventeen of all races was 16.9 percent and for girls eighteen to nineteen it was 14.9 percent. Only 5 percent of doula-supported moms delivered low-birth-weight babies, compared to 13 percent of teens who gave birth in Georgia. Similar programs in Denver, Indianapolis, Fort Worth, and Brooklyn are currently gathering data on low- and very-low-birth-weight babies to see if the trend holds.

Based on these compelling findings, the U.S. Congress for the first time appropriated $1.5 million in the 2008 budget to replicate and expand the community-based doula project nationally. Senator Dick Durbin and then-senator Barack Obama, both Democrats of Illinois, and Bob Casey, a Pennsylvania Democrat, were key supporters.

We'll refer a number of times in our book to research cataloged by the Cochrane Collaboration, whose story deserves a special mention. In the 1970s, British epidemiologist Archie Cochrane declared that doctors should make decisions based on the best research available. He created a ranking of medical specialties according to whether they made use of scientific evidence, and found that obstetrics came in last. He also analyzed a collection of the available studies on maternity care, the first such review of its kind. This led others to create the Cochrane Collaboration shortly after his death, which has grown into a renowned, independent, and nonprofit center for the review of studies in dozens of medical specialties, and can be visited at www.cochrane.org.

Regarding best medical procedures, the American College of Obstetricians and Gynecologists publishes "practice bulletins" (or articles) to guide doctors in their decision-making. In March 2006, the *American Journal of Obstetrics & Gynecology* published a study that reviewed all fifty-five of ACOG's current practice bulletins, calling these articles "perhaps the most influential publications for clinicians involved with obstetric and gynecological care."

The study concluded that "among 438 recommendations made by ACOG, less than one third [23 percent] are based on good and consistent scientific evidence."

Some widely used procedures, not supported by evidence, appear to hinder normal labor, while others simply haven't been tested yet to prove whether they are harmful or beneficial. Obstetric research is complex, and no one doctor, midwife, or doula has all the answers. Also, no two practitioners follow the exact same guidelines. Remember, though, that you deserve respectful conversation with your caregivers about any questions you may have. You're entitled to participate in making your own best decisions, taking into consideration your doctor's advice, information from reliable books and Internet sources, and your personal knowledge of your family.

## CAN DOULAS PREVENT ALL INTERVENTIONS?

Using a doula may be *the best thing you can do as an individual pregnant woman* to help improve today's labor and delivery care and the options available to you in the hospital.

A doula is appropriate whether you desire a completely natural childbirth or know that you plan to use an epidural. Childbirth Connection reports that more than one-third of women who take birthing classes do so in hopes of preparing for a drug-free labor. And there are sizable numbers of women in another category: those who plan to wait and see what actually happens in labor before deciding whether to use pain medication.

Be prepared, though: in reality, the use of epidurals and other medical procedures is currently very high. Without a doula, epidurals are used in the U.S. by approximately 85 percent or more of first-time mothers, with rates going down slightly for women having their second or subsequent baby. Canadians use anesthesia 53 percent of the time, according to the Canadian Institute for Health Information, as do 34 percent of the British, according to the National Health Service.

The use of cesarean section in the United States is at its highest rate ever, now at nearly one in three births; similar rates are reported by nations including Australia, Brazil, Canada, Chile, Greece, Italy, Taiwan, and Turkey.

There is wide variation in the use of obstetric interventions, which may depend on what region of the country you live in, your particular hospital, and whether you choose a midwife or doctor as your primary care provider. (For example, the use of episiotomy, a cut made by doctors to enlarge the vagina, is at a relatively low rate of 5 to 10 percent in the Boston area, where the authors of this book live. In other parts of the U.S., though—even in other parts of our state—it is still routinely used 25 percent or more of the time.)

### ❧ ASK YOUR DOCTOR NOW ❧

Be sure to ask your doctor or midwife to provide you with the statistics of procedures used at your hospital, including the rates of natural childbirth, epidurals, and cesareans. This may be one of the most important questions that you ask, which will help you know what to expect of your caregivers' approach.

There is also variation in the effect that each doula is able to have. Some women with labor assistants experience fewer interventions than others, which may be partly attributable to the doula's experience level. Also, research shows that when a doula is self-employed, mothers have fewer interventions than when a doula is employed by the hospital.

Scientists began studying doulas in the 1970s, and since that time maternity care has undergone dramatic changes. Hospitals did not make epidurals available to the majority of mothers thirty years ago, and 5 percent of births were cesareans, a mere one-sixth of their current rate. Today, epidurals and cesareans have become everyday events. Doulas still impact the rates of these interventions. But the high rates of interventions also impact doulas. Studies report that it can be harder (though not impossible) for doulas to lower the use of medical procedures at hospitals where rates are highest.

Doulas reduce interventions—but they have not eliminated them. The trend toward heavy use of obstetric interventions means it's possible that when a doula is present, these procedures may still be used, even on mothers who expect not to need them. We encourage you to get prepared for the normal, high intensity of a labor without interventions, and we'll be talking more about how to do that. We also encourage you to get prepared for the possibility that medical procedures may be used, *even if that is not your plan.*

If you wish to have natural childbirth, doulas truly are useful in their role as pain-relievers and for their effect of reducing interventions. If you plan to use an epidural, labor can still be emotionally charged, filled with unexpected events and decision-making, and a doula can help navigate this.

When medical procedures are used that were unplanned, the support of a doula may be needed most. A doula can support you in making difficult choices with more confidence, to get through frightening moments without feeling alone, and to focus on the joys of giving birth even in the midst of stressful circumstances. Complicated births, interventions, and cesareans can sometimes have lasting stressful effects, including increased chances of postpartum depression, more challenges with breastfeeding, more need for help at home with the new baby, or even symptoms of trauma. Be aware of this possibility so you can seek out family or professional help to turn this situation around if needed.

In perspective, the November 2008 issue of the *American Journal of Obstetrics & Gynecology* looked at more than forty aspects of labor and delivery management based on scientific evidence, and recommended doula care itself as "one of the most effective interventions."

## WHAT TO EXPECT IN THE LABOR WARD: BEING A GUEST OF THE HOSPITAL

Most women in industrialized countries give birth in hospitals, which means you are a guest on someone else's terrain. Understanding this dynamic can help you to be better prepared for your experience there.

Your hosts (the hospital staff) will explain how to make yourself comfortable, by showing you where to find items like pillows and blankets and how to get telephone service. And they'll also explain limits on your behavior, such as controversial practices in many hospitals that deny women in labor food and drink.

You may find yourself moved by the kindness of your labor and delivery providers, or frustrated if they seem to overlook your needs during a time of great vulnerability. Having your baby in a hospital, you may be overjoyed with your birth, disappointed or upset by today's care, or plainly satisfied with no regrets.

The members of your personal support team are also guests inside the hospital, including your mate if you're partnered, your family and friends, and your doula. Some hospitals welcome as many members of your support system as you wish to invite. Other hospitals strictly limit the number of guests you may bring, without the option of having anyone other than one family member and your doula with you.

During certain medical procedures, such as the insertion of an epidural or in the event of a cesarean section, doctors may ask your support people to exit the room for part of the procedure. Some doctors permit one family member as well as your doula to be present for a cesarean, while others permit only one support person into the operating room.

As guests of the hospital, you and your loved ones are agreeing to generally respect the customs and limits set by your hosts—even though this may mean compromising some of your wishes. And although a doula is your advocate, she's still obligated to show sensitivity to the rules of the hospital.

On the other hand, your doctor or midwife, nurse, and the hospital staff are hired by you. As their employer you have the right to request that your preferences be followed, or at a minimum, considered and discussed. No procedure can lawfully be done without your consent, except in case of very rare emergencies. When necessary, you can ask for a second opinion, or that your caregiver be replaced by someone who is a better match for you.

(If you want the most control and the least restrictions on your behavior and that of your support team, learn about the option of giving birth at home or in a freestanding birth center. When birthing at home, the midwife or doctor is a guest in your domain, where rates of complications may actually be lower. The need to negotiate could still arise, but you'll have the most freedom in your own home. For more information, see the 2002 book *Birth Your Way: Choosing Birth at Home or in a Birth Center* by childbirth expert Sheila Kitzinger.)

## WILL YOUR DOCTOR ACTUALLY BE THERE FOR LABOR?

Who will actually be your medical provider on the day you give birth? Many parents are unaware that in a hospital, doctors and midwives often work on rotation, with each caregiver in a group covering only one day of the week in labor and delivery. If this is the case with your provider, it's likely that you may be cared for in labor by someone you have never (or barely) met before, as reported by at least one in three mothers in a national survey.

Some midwives and doctors still do attend the births of their own patients. When they learn you are in labor, they may be busy seeing other patients in their office, and they may communicate instructions by phone to a nurse who is caring for you on the labor and delivery floor. Many doctors spend only a few minutes at a time with women during their labors, and are not available to give you their undivided attention until the final hour of your birth. Midwives in hospitals sometimes focus on providing more guidance during labor itself, although they also may need to leave your room or not be available during much of labor.

So what are doctors and midwives doing while you are in labor and they are not in the room with you? They are probably checking on and delivering other women who are in labor at the same time as you. They may have a dozen or more mothers to visit in the postpartum ward who've given birth in the last several days. They may be sleeping in an on-call room during a long shift, or simply waiting in a staff room until they are notified that a patient needs them. In general, obstetricians are not available to take on the role of your labor support provider.

You'll receive more attention from your nurse than your doctor in the United States and Canada. Many hospitals assign one nurse to every two mothers in labor. Nurses typically visit you a couple of times an hour to take vital signs for you and your baby, including listening to heartbeats, taking blood pressure, and taking your temperature, as well as drawing blood and administering drugs if needed, and then documenting their work. (Countries including Austria and the United Kingdom do not use maternity nurses; there, midwives are responsible for all of these clinical tasks.)

Some nurses enjoy providing labor coaching and support, while others take a more hands-off approach. Because of the ratio of one nurse to several mothers in labor, it is usually not possible for a nurse to provide undivided attention to you in labor. Research shows that mothers assume their nurses will spend approximately 53 percent of their time providing labor support, yet in reality less than 10 percent of nurses' time is spent in this way. Most of their time is spent on medical care.

Doctors, midwives, and nurses commonly work in shifts that last from eight to twenty-four hours, at which point they will hand over your care to the next provider. In a teaching hospital, the turnover may be even greater, and a completely different doctor might check on you every couple of hours. If you are having your first baby, *expect* to be cared for by at least two shifts of nurses and doctors, and possibly three or four shifts. While you're pregnant, ask your doctor or midwife if they will attend your birth or if they work on rotation with other providers, so you know what to anticipate. Also ask if they will provide any coaching throughout labor, or mainly just be present at the end for delivery.

As you've probably figured out by now, using a doula helps fill in the many gaps in coverage that are a result of doctors, midwives, and nurses being on rotation, caring for multiple patients in labor, performing clinical tasks and paperwork, and changing shifts.

## RETURNING BIRTH TO WOMEN

Women around the world and throughout time have known how to take care of each other in birth. They've shown each other the best positions for comfort in labor, they've used nurturing touch and repeated soothing words, and they've literally held each other up when it's needed the most. Today doulas are helping revive this essential tradition. (And in the process, they're helping lower the need for drugs in labor.) Remember—a birth doula *is* a form of pain relief.

I come from a family of African immigrants. When my labor got really strong, my own mother held me in her arms almost the entire time. She whispered again and again, "Have courage, have courage." My husband, doula, and doctor were there, too. For three days of early labor, my doula helped me with positions and breathing techniques, and she also listened on the fourth day when I needed to decide whether to use narcotics. My mom was able to be such a natural "doula" too—she knew just what to say in the toughest moments.

—Carine, 36, journalist, mother of three

In large, multicultural cities, doulas sometimes have the opportunity to work with a clientele that hails from every sub-continent on the globe. Watching women give birth, you can see that what our culture taught us greatly influences whether we expect to be able to handle labor. A mother originally from South America describes the attitudes about birth in her native country:

While I was pregnant, I was sitting at home with my two doulas and my aunt. We were talking about what labor would feel like. My aunt said, "Oh, you'll feel kind of strange all day, and then it hurts for a half hour, and you have the baby." That was what she learned growing up!

When the day came I had back labor, and if you've heard that it's harder than regular labor, it's true. But my boyfriend and doulas gave me a lot of support to hang in there. I felt overwhelmed for a couple of hours—not much longer than my aunt said—and then I was ready to deliver.

—Marta, 22, student, mother of one

Doulas help mothers learn what to expect in birth. They tell women the truth about the intensity of labor and help them discover their strength. They educate their clients, and they do research on whatever topics their clients might need: from exercises to turn a breech baby, to which doctors in town can deliver twins by vaginal birth, to finding volunteers who provide home visits to new mothers.

Compared to a decade ago, many more families have at least heard about doulas. But still, a labor assistant's services are not yet an automatic part of maternity care. Parents often must look for it. However, doula care should not be seen as an extra service. Rather, it's something that has been removed from the birthing room, and advocates for mothers and babies are working to bring it back. Without skilled labor support, the experience of pain increases, as do routine interventions and complications during birth.

Today families often need to search around to find their doula, but it's well worth the effort it might take you. There are currently thousands of doulas listed on the Internet, on referral lists at hospitals and birth centers, and elsewhere. Their services are paid for by you directly, by your insurance or government funds such as Medicaid, by your hospital or birth center, or offered by community volunteers.

Congratulations for discovering the wonderful option of doulas, and the leading-edge knowledge about birth that they have to share with the world.

### ⟢ WHAT'S IN A NAME? ⟣

This book, *The Doula Guide to Birth,* focuses mainly on the ways a birth doula can assist you. Although they may sound related, the practitioners known as birth doulas, postpartum doulas, and midwives do not offer the same services. Their roles are distinguished below.

### BIRTH DOULA

A birth doula specializes in providing one-on-one physical and emotional comfort during labor. She gives continuous labor support, usually without breaks or shift changes. She is not the one to deliver the baby. Other common terms for a birth doula include: labor assistant, labor support provider.

### POSTPARTUM DOULA

A postpartum doula is not usually present at the birth. She specializes in helping the new family at home after the baby is born. Her duties can include baby care, breastfeeding support, daytime or overnight care, and household tasks such as cooking and laundry.

### MIDWIFE

A midwife has more advanced training than a birth doula, and she can be your primary care provider and deliver your baby, instead of a doctor. Midwives usually train for several years in a university or nursing school in order to become caregivers in hospitals, or by the apprentice method in order to supervise births at home.

# 2

# FOR FATHERS, PARTNERS, AND OTHER LOVED ONES

B irth, despite its intimate nature, has always been a social event. Traditionally, relatives and friends helped the mother through labor. These days families are far-flung, and the very notion of "family" is in flux.

A pregnant woman might be supported by her husband, boyfriend, lesbian partner, her own mother, another relative, or friends. She may also have the company of the baby's father with whom she's no longer romantically involved, a sperm donor father, or the baby's adoptive parents. While the laboring woman will be the obvious focus of attention, her observers and outside supporters may require help and guidance for themselves as well.

Women in Western cultures today usually labor with the father of their child by their side, and for most couples, the experience brings them together in powerful ways, forging their first bonds as a family. This chapter will offer fathers, partners, and loved ones some strategies for fully engaging in birth so the experience will be both positive and memorable, along with making the most of a doula's assistance.

## FATHERHOOD

Expectant fathers, taking on what the anthropologist Richard Reed describes as a "sympathetic" process of gestation, might stop smoking, reduce their drinking, drive less aggressively, or buy life insurance. But for most men, fatherhood doesn't begin in earnest until the moment you actually see your newborn. You might be elated, anxious, or awed, but most new dads say they also feel a deep, biological sense of responsibility and protectiveness. The birth of your child can also be tinged with fear, as well as the sobering realization that you have finally and irreversibly become an adult.

For others, having a child is the fulfillment of a fantasy harbored quietly for many years.

> From a young age, I dreamed of becoming a father——I literally had dreams about what my daughter would look like——but I never discussed it with my male friends. When she was born, it was like a part of me finally got a chance to come out into the light.
>
> ——Jack, 41, history teacher, father of three

### Out With the Cigars, and Into the Fire

Ever since the early 1900s, when birth moved out of homes and into hospitals, fathers have been trying to figure out their role.

In the late 1940s, American obstetrician-gynecologist Dr. Robert Bradley developed what he called Husband-Coached Childbirth, later to become known as the Bradley Method, which was truly revolutionary in its envisioning of fathers on the front lines of birth. The husband acted as the birthing "coach," a role of critical importance for the new family. In 1951, Dr. Fernand Lamaze introduced a method of natural childbirth in France that incorporated techniques he had observed in Russia. This method, best known for its regimented breathing techniques, was intended to trigger a physiological response that helped move the birthing process along. It was introduced in the U.S. in the late 1950s and widely embraced two decades later, when fathers finally won the right to be in delivery rooms with their wives during birth. Lamaze fathers also played a central role, demonstrating the intense breathing sequences for the laboring mothers to mimic.

Today, the Lamaze organization has moved away from its strict breathing techniques, and the notion of "coaching" a laboring woman has broadened.

We invite you to approach birth without a rigid script. Know that your presence and ability to listen and respond moment by moment to all of the emotional and physical manifestations of labor will contribute to the process in profound ways. Just like the laboring mom must relax and surrender herself in order to birth, so too partners, loved ones, and particularly fathers may have to let go of trying to control the process.

During pregnancy, doulas work closely with both you and your partner to point out how each of you is contributing and how to enhance that teamwork. Well before the birth, the doula will begin to get a sense of the couple's dynamic, stressors, and hopes and fears about birth.

Fathers should know that a doula is a professional labor assistant who offers comfort measures and emotional support to both of you throughout labor. She will not replace you, nor will she provide medical advice or clinical care in the hospital. Her job is to be a constant presence during labor, and offer, among other things, techniques to deal with the intensity of contractions, emotional assurance, backup if you need to take a break or check on an older child, and guidance to help the process unfold in the ways you and your partner envision.

George, a builder in his late thirties, says that with support from a doula, he was able to overcome his apprehension and marvel at his wife Erica's power during the birth of their son. Erica had always been known as the "catastrophizer" in the family. But throughout labor, she used self-hypnosis techniques that allowed her to remain calm and strong for hours. Her doula, Marianne, was instrumental in helping Erica maintain that relaxed, self-assured state. She whispered into Erica's ear and kept her room quiet and softly lit. George says before the birth, he was secretly worried about Erica's ability to cope, but that the birth of his daughter was so peaceful and moving that his anxiety simply disappeared. Two years later, the couple invited their mothers to watch their second child's birth. "The whole process was like a pride thing for me," George says. "We had told people how well Erica did the first time, but the second time we had witnesses. I was so happy to have an audience for the event—I kept saying, 'See how great she is.'"

Studies have documented fathers' stress levels surging at various points throughout labor. That's not surprising, since, apart from the intensity of the experience, fathers sometimes feel torn between different roles. They want to support their partners, which takes a good deal of focus, but they also feel responsible for taking on other jobs, like negotiating with hospital staff and advocating for their partners' needs. Studies show that dads feel less pressure to advocate when doulas are present.

Having a doula can free you up to connect with your wife or partner and share one of life's most transformative experiences. As one father put it, "Witnessing birth made me feel more connected to the human race."

Such raw emotionality can be dampened by a hospital culture that might seem impersonal and foreign, particularly for first-time parents. If you've never witnessed labor, you might worry that what your partner is enduring is too painful or that something has gone wrong. Doulas are adept at reassuring loved ones that what they are watching is normal or, if it isn't, at calmly explaining what is happening.

James, a nineteen-year-old musician who learned about doulas through a hospital program, was eager to play a central role in his first child's birth and took a number of classes to prepare for the event. He and his girlfriend learned special relaxation techniques to ease the pain of labor. But, he says, he forgot the techniques when the time came and found that the doula offered much more practical help, and acted as a sort of narrator throughout the process. "One of the best parts about having a doula was when my girlfriend was uncomfortable, or in pain, or feeling frustrated because it seemed nothing was going on, I knew the doula knew what was going on. I knew if either of us had any questions, there was someone to turn to, and that relieved so much stress."

Unexpected surgery or a particularly long, painful labor can throw even the most calm and grounded person into a high-stress state. One twenty-eight-year-old father, recalling the birth of his daughter, says his own fear was greatly reduced knowing that his wife had another powerful ally:

> I was anxious, for myself and my wife, and saw her struggling physically through a very difficult labor. It was painful, literally and figuratively, to

> witness. Long and hard for her, and for all of us
> present. The nurses kept telling me I should encour-
> age my wife to get the epidural, but I knew she didn't
> want it. Our doula was very calming in her manner
> and mood—she protected my wife and steadied
> her, and helped her give birth to Lily just how we'd
> envisioned.

As fathers and partners, your touch, supportive words, and expressions of love help birth along, triggering the release of the hormone oxytocin, which stimulates contractions. Finding the space to make this connection—in a highly charged environment, where your lover is on full display and at her most vulnerable—is a central challenge of birth.

> I am a fairly involved guy, but at birth, I was super-
> involved. I remember Chantal was pushing and the
> blood was everywhere and the midwife said, "Why
> don't you start massaging her perineum [the open-
> ing of her birth canal]," so I did. And she was groan-
> ing and I was massaging and suddenly the head was
> right there, and I was really in something of an al-
> tered state and I heard a voice say, "It's a girl," and I
> was giddy and I thought, "My God, it's a girl!"
>
> —Elijah, 32, sculptor, father of two

The emotions that arise during birth may surprise you. The experience could stir up old memories, perhaps painful, of your own father or experiences as a child. For this reason, it's important to articulate your fears as well as your hopes with your partner and doula before birth.

———————

Research shows when fathers connect with their partners and newborns through labor and birth, healthier parental bonds develop. A 2007 analysis funded by the National Institutes of Health found that fathers who were more involved throughout pregnancy, including participating in prenatal care, childbirth classes, and being present at the birth, were more likely to participate in child-rearing and engaged in a higher level of cognitively stimulating activities with their young children. These fathers also showed more warmth and nurturing behavior toward their children and provided more hands-on physical care, such as changing diapers and giving baths.

To facilitate this early involvement, doulas typically meet with the couple in person several times before birth (and frequently by e-mail and on the phone throughout the pregnancy) to encourage teamwork, help alleviate fears, and answer questions that come up. (*How will I know whether she should get an epidural? How will we know when labor is really starting? Can I help catch the baby as it is being born?*) Doulas will ask directly about you, the father, to learn about your needs and how you want to participate. One father said his doula called him after a meeting with him and his wife to ask whether he had any questions to ask privately.

As the father or partner, you may be skittish about hiring or using a doula because you might feel you are being replaced as the lead support person. Perhaps you are uncomfortable with the prospect of an outsider's presence at such an intimate event. But most fathers report that in retrospect, those worries were unfounded. Studies show fathers participate *more* when a doula is present. Moreover, with doctors, nurses, and possibly several others in the room, birth is not usually a quiet, low-key affair. In fact, in order to help protect the couple's intimacy and shield them from chatter, background noise, and other intrusions, a priority for the doula is to make the room as calm and peaceful as possible.

## NO LONGER LOVERS

When expectant parents are estranged or struggling over whether to remain a couple, a new approach by the professional support team is warranted, says Elizabeth Davis, a respected trainer of midwives based in California. She says in order to keep some of the bonds of the fractured family intact, it's critical to have the father or partner present at the birth (unless, of course, abuse is involved). "I've observed, particularly men having their first child, they don't understand there's a baby until the moment they see the baby—they don't connect with the baby until they see it—that's the powerful and unexpectedly emotional moment for the father."

If the father wishes to be present and the mother permits it, doulas will encourage his involvement. This might require more conversations before birth about the laboring woman's needs in this situation. For instance, a mom might ask the dad to be present for the labor, but not pushing, when she wants more privacy. Or she might ask him not to be present for the whole labor but to wait until the end. The dad might need extra help coping with strong emotions like loneliness and loss. It may be helpful for him to ask a friend or relative of his to remain in the waiting room as his support person. (However, a new romantic partner is probably not the right person to do this.)

## LESBIAN PARTNERS

Lesbian families face unique challenges during pregnancy and labor. Though progress has been made by the gay community, homophobia and bias still exist, including in the realm of birth and parenting.

Birthing books and other materials more often than not address "fathers" and "husbands." One expectant mother said that in most of the standard childbirth literature, nothing spoke to her as a gay partner of a woman about to give birth. She said her doula was able to pull together various information that was relevant to her situation. "Most of the books for partners were written for the man ignorant of the process—the caveman approach, where the men were clueless and the women were hormonal and irrational and I kept asking myself, 'Who am I in this book?' I'm not a pregnant woman, but I'm not a man. Having an actual person who 'got it,' who could talk about how it would be emotionally, was extremely helpful."

Over the years, books for gay families have occasionally appeared; our favorite is *The New Essential Guide to Lesbian Conception, Pregnancy & Birth,* by midwife and fertility expert Stephanie Brill.

Many lesbian mothers are open with their care providers about their orientation, but some are still hesitant to come out, and choose to refer to their partner as their friend. Since the legal rights of partners vary by state and country, lesbian couples generally have to arrange in advance whether the non-birthing woman can make medical decisions for her partner.

Emotionally, lesbian co-mothers sometimes feel extra pressure to fill the role of doula by themselves because they are female.

"You have such a different situation when women are to-gether," Ms. Davis, the California midwife, says. "Women are very aware of each other's hormones and serve to mirror and heighten one another's awareness. When a woman wants to help, that is to be encouraged."

But, she says, it's easier for a lesbian partner to go into "lover" mode with the birthing mother, meaning the partner often pushes aside her own feelings of fatigue, anxiety, and any residual conflicts from her own experience giving birth, if she has done so. The doula must keep an eye on the lesbian partner, who might want a time-out but not recognize it.

"Women feel compelled to keep going—to go beyond themselves, we do it all the time," Ms. Davis says. "We nurture beyond our capacity and overlook our own needs."

Rose, a gay woman whose partner endured a tough labor with twins, describes the relief she felt when she realized it was okay to take a break and relinquish the role of coach in order to feel her own unsteadiness and fear:

> I'm squeamish, and I was nervous about what it would be like to see my partner in a lot of pain, worried about my ability to be a rock and be there the whole time. I had my own performance anxiety and having a doula and others to support me was great. I would get really overwhelmed with emotions and have to leave the room but that was okay since I knew Megan was surrounded by support and she wouldn't feel alone.

## GRANDMOTHERS

Expectant parents caught up in the excitement of birth can be self-absorbed, and understandably so. But they often overlook a profound phenomenon happening as their baby is born: their own mothers are undergoing a complex transition to becoming grandmothers.

The British anthropologist Sheila Kitzinger, commenting on this little-discussed transformation, writes:

> Being turned into a grandmother—a choice you did not yourself make in any active way—propels you into territory yet unmapped. You are on marginal land, picking your way over ground that lies between motherhood and being a respected "tribal elder." Just as with your first day of school or your first period, the first time you had sex or committed yourself to another human being, when

you were pregnant and after the birth of the baby, becoming a grandmother constitutes a life passage . . . When a woman is expecting a baby there are books, magazines, classes—ways of preparing herself for the challenge ahead . . . When she becomes a grandmother, there is nothing like this.

In many ways, there is nothing more natural than a mother supporting her own daughter giving birth. Yet grandmothers may have their own conflicts and memories associated with this passage. A lot has changed in a generation of maternity care, and it is helpful for expectant grandmothers to educate themselves. *Attending Your Grandchild's Birth: A Guide for Grandparents,* by Carolynn Bauer Zorn is one book that can begin to orient grandparents to the various technologies and current issues in childbirth. Grandmothers may simply need an outlet if they are anxious, and they could approach the doula for help with this. Oftentimes, grandmothers can read their own children quite well, and may make important contributions to the experience.

One grandmother who watched her daughter give birth remembers feeling surprised and displaced when she learned her daughter hired a doula: "I said, 'What are you talking about?' I didn't know what a doula was. I come from pretty humble beginnings—women didn't work—and here my kid says, 'I'm hiring a doula.'" But when the birth finally happened, the grandmother, age fifty-two, was in awe. "I had two children, and when I look back on my births—the pain, the screaming—it was amazing to sit there and watch my daughter with the doula whispering in her ear—just wonderful to watch her give birth and not scream in pain. We were quiet, the lights were down low, and it was really peaceful."

Another grandmother, after watching her daughter-in-law give birth, said:

> I gave birth back in the day when you were knocked out and woke up with a bundle all clean and swaddled. Consequently, I never witnessed a birth except on television. To see her go through that whole process calmly with the doula, and to see my grandson being born, was most definitely a highlight of my life which I will never forget.

## THE NEW NUCLEAR FAMILY

In addition to the partner, a doula helps guide other loved ones who may not have attended birthing classes or have experience with birth. For example, some pregnant women ask a sister or female friend to be at their births, even if these other women supporters have not been pregnant. Less typically, an important male friend or family member is included.

A gay man and sperm donor, Emmanuel, says he was surprised by his own emotional reaction to the birth of his daughter. One of the high points, he says, was when the doula asked him to hold up a taut sheet so the laboring mom could pull on it and get herself into a more comfortable position. "I wasn't just a passive witness, I was an active participant," he says. "I became an anchor for her and at one point our eyes locked and she was pushing and I was using all my strength, and it allowed her partner to be with her and hold her." Emmanuel says as a gay man, he never imagined watching the birth of his own child. "It's a gift and it will probably never happen again," he says. "Having held her as a newborn and having been in her glow, now I look at children with much more compassion. Everything feels more precious and tender."

## ADOPTION

Felicity, a doula who helped a young woman, Denise, through labor before she placed her baby for adoption, said that the experience was one of the most emotional she has witnessed as a doula. Felicity says she frequently acted as a messenger, delivering updates to the adoptive family in the hall. When Denise's own mother arrived and questioned her daughter's decision to give the baby up, Felicity says she tried to shield Denise by letting the older woman vent about her conflicting feelings. "I became her mother's doula, too," Felicity says. After a long labor, Denise ended up having a C-section. For her part, Denise says she simply could not have endured such an emotional time without Felicity's help. "She was my primary support person," Denise says. "No matter what happened, I knew I wouldn't be alone." (For more information on these issues, please also see the section "Doula Specialty: Adoption and Surrogacy" in chapter 5.)

## THE BABY'S SIBLINGS

Having one or more older siblings present at birth can truly bring a family together, provided that the mother feels comfortable and excited by the prospect. If you are considering this option, there are a few things to address. The most important question is whether the presence of an older sibling will be a distraction for the laboring mother. The other critical issue is whether the older child really wants to be there. If you decide to do it, make sure the older child is prepared; read him age-appropriate books about birth and talk to him about how birth might unfold. Also, make sure there's a designated adult whose sole responsibility is to care for the child during the entire labor and someone who understands the child can change his or her mind anytime.

Amanda, a doula whose four-year-old son was present for the birth of his sister, says the experience gave the older child a much deeper understanding of family, and a sense that he and his baby sister came into the world in a special and magical way.

Another mother, Alana, had planned for her son to be at her home birth, but now says she's glad he ended up at a friend's house until after the baby was born. "I think I would have been too distracted," she says, "and feeling responsible for him when I should have been concentrating on labor."

## A DOULA'S PLACE

The doula is available to offer assistance and guidance to whoever steps into the birthing circle. She demonstrates labor positions in which moms can lean against their partners or loved ones. She praises the mother in labor, which helps partners feel less shy about saying loving things during birth, too. She clears the room if the couple needs time for snuggling as a way to help labor progress. (A stalled labor may often be hastened by the release of hormones associated with physical intimacy.)

If the support people need tasks, a doula can dole them out. Many partners need guidance about how to offer effective forms of massage and touch when their mate is in pain. Doulas can remind loved ones when it is time to feed the mother and themselves throughout the long hours of labor. If a partner needs to check on an older child or give updates to nervous relatives or simply take a break, a doula will remain in the labor room.

Most partners and moms benefit from closeness in labor, and a doula helps facilitate this by creating an environment of calm and security. Occasionally, though, a partner is struggling with deeper challenges that he or she cannot easily resolve, such as depression or a sense of being overwhelmed. In these cases, a doula may be able to reassure the partner that he or she is allowed to participate—or not participate—to the degree that brings the most comfort and the least added stress to the birth.

Whether a women labors with her partner only or she brings others—a photographer, acupuncturist, sperm donor, or belly-dance instructor to help demonstrate traditional movements that may ease labor pain—it is a doula's job to help harmonize the group's efforts. There can be advantages to enlarging the circle of close relations who will be present at birth. A sense of intimacy can actually be increased when a mom or couple has the support of several loved ones, rather than being surrounded only by unfamiliar medical personnel.

Some women are unsure of whom to bring to their births or they feel pressured by people who ask to attend. Remember, the laboring woman shouldn't have to worry about seating arrangements or whether everyone has snacks. She should not be put in a position of trying to live up to other people's expectations. One obstetrician commented that even during childbirth, women tend to focus on making everyone else feel OK. "Even in labor we try to please people, whether it's to be quiet, or to be passive, or to be good and do what we're told," she said. The mother needs to be able to let all of these expectations go no matter who else is in the room.

Some mothers do prefer to invite a larger crowd, especially teens, some home-birth moms, and immigrants or residents of countries with different customs than those found in Western hospitals. Talk with your doula about how to decide whom to include.

## MANAGING EXPECTATIONS

Many partners describe how their expectations of birth simply don't match up with the real thing.

A study of fourteen first-time fathers in the *Journal of Nurse-Midwifery* found that men's pre-birth notions of what labor would be like were far from reality—particularly if labor was long and progress was slow. These men reported that as labor got more intense "they learned that it required more work than they anticipated." For example, some of the men supported their wives in a squatting position for a long time while others offered massages. "They were amazed at how tiresome this became," the study says. Some of the men said they were also discouraged that many of the coping techniques they learned did not work. In addition, all of the men said that when hospital staff did not answer their questions fully, come when called, or announced plans for unanticipated interventions, they felt more anxiety and "as a result could not concentrate fully on their wives."

A fifty-three-year-old lawyer and first-time father explains:

> While my partner was pregnant, we spent a lot of time talking with our doula about what to expect during labor. There was no way, though, that I could really imagine the birth until it actually happened. It was a super-intense experience, but I watched our doula and midwife during the labor, and they were calm and acting as if everything was normal. That allowed me to relax as best I could, and go with what was happening.

## SUPPORT FOR THE UNEXPECTED

When birth takes an unexpected turn, tension can spike and loved ones may find themselves caught off guard. One couple expecting their third child had prepared for a non-medicated birth with a doula and a quiet atmosphere. What they got was the opposite. After laboring for two days with many medical attempts to hasten the birth, a new obstetrician came on duty and told Sarah she needed an immediate C-section, something she had described as "her worst nightmare." Her husband, Donald, recalls his frustration being stuck in a precarious position: torn between trusting the doctor while knowing that surgery would be disappointing and scary for his wife. He didn't know whether to talk Sarah into the C-section or nudge the doctor to let her labor more. Donald said he couldn't have handled all that responsibility without their doula's encouragement and acknowledgment that the surgery would be OK. The doula asked the doctor to allow her into the operating room to provide emotional support for both parents, and the baby was born healthy. Sarah was sad about the experience, but instead of trying to "fix" it, Donald and the doula together let her grieve and move on.

"It didn't go the way we'd hoped," Donald said. "But it was the birth we had, and by the time we took the baby home, the crisis atmosphere had faded and we quickly fell in love."

However birth unfolds for you, it will likely be a transforming experience. We encourage you to engage the process in the way that fits you best. Know that simply by listening and responding to the laboring woman, your presence will benefit the new mother, the newborn, and you. And remember that your doula's goal is to help create an environment in which everyone present—father, family members, or other supporters—can participate as fully as possible.

# 3

# LABOR, THE HARDEST WORK YOU'LL EVER LOVE?

*Those last few hours were incredibly hard for me,
but it really was the best day of my life.*

—Tanisha, 33, homemaker, mother of two

Giving birth is likely to be the most trying work you'll ever do in the course of a normal life. And yet, mothers throughout time have accomplished this heroic act and come through it feeling many things: relieved, shaken, amazed, grateful, or thrilled, to name a few.

We believe the most helpful way to prepare for birth is to have a realistic view of how charged and challenging this event can be. Yes, labor is often very athletic, intensely hard work. It is involuntary, unstoppable, and takes every ounce of your attention and energy, mentally and physically. Luckily for first-time mothers, it also tends to be a gradual process, with many built-in breaks. Your future labors may have fewer breaks, but will usually be much shorter.

While it's important to be realistically aware that labor may well be the toughest thing you'll ever do, it's also vital to be aware that you can do it, and that it stretches you to your limits in such a way that you will find out how strong, not weak, you are. That knowledge is what women relied on for centuries to give birth, and it's the most effective and encouraging approach we know of.

So how does labor unfold?

The basics: women usually describe it starting as a strong, rhythmic tightening and hardening of their belly area, or a dull cramping that is not painful in the beginning. Every few hours, these contractions become more powerful, and eventually evolve into sensations often described as painful and intense. This intensity increases until you near the end of labor; you may feel overwhelmed and consumed at this point. However, this is also the shortest part of labor, known as *transition,* and generally lasts for only about an hour, until it is time to completely push your baby out of your body.

Labor pain is muscular, like the pain of running a marathon, to which it has often been compared. (In fact, one result of childbirth is that athletes who've gone through it become faster at their sport.) It is not the pain of breaking a bone, or being cut, hit, stung, scalded—or heartbroken. The pain of labor is felt in the uterus, the same muscle involved in producing an orgasm or menstrual cramps; labor takes these sensations to their ultimate strength.

> When my wife was in labor, our doula suggested
> she sigh and moan to relieve her pain. At first, my
> wife made a few soft noises. During hard labor,

though, she was moaning loudly, about ten times with every contraction.

The midwife came in and asked my wife how she felt. My wife said she felt good, and that after she moaned one or two times, she knew she could make it through the rest of that contraction. That was great for me to hear—her labor looked overwhelming to me, but she was actually doing fine, and it was a relief for me to understand she wasn't being pushed past what she could really handle.

—Stewart, 28, marketing consultant, father of one

Nearly all women have been heard to say "I can't do it" at the end of labor. They do not actually know what their reserves of strength look like yet, because no other situation in life has tested them like labor. But that strength is indeed there. With each phase of labor, the mother adjusts physically and emotionally to the increased sensations. She sees she is not dying or being harmed, and that she can, in fact, do this. Even when she says, "I can't do it," she is likely to be venting about the great effort her body is making for the first time in her life—not necessarily asking for drugs. It is normal to cry out briefly (and loudly) from stress at the end of labor. This cry is usually a sign that the hardest threshold has been crossed, and the baby will arrive soon.

---

Although this may be your first baby, you've probably already had a preview of some of the sensations of labor. Starting in the first trimester of pregnancy, all women begin to have Braxton-Hicks contractions, or practice contractions in which the uterus exercises itself by tightening and releasing, though they may not be noticeable until late in pregnancy. (It would be wonderful if all the muscles of our bodies would exercise themselves like this, without us having to think about it.) Labor contractions work the same way as Braxton-Hicks contractions, only they are *significantly stronger*. They're usually intense enough that you will be able to say, "These are definitely different than what I felt throughout pregnancy."

If you have had menstrual cramps, you also have a sense of what labor may feel like. Some women and girls experience menstrual cramps as a mild ache across their belly; other women have felt extremely painful menstrual cramps which consumed all their attention and interrupted their normal activities. Women with previous infertility, endometriosis, or other pelvic pain conditions are especially likely to have had cramping powerful enough to be described as labor-like.

While many women characterize labor as painful, some mothers have described it otherwise. In his book *Painless Childbirth,* Dr. Lamaze wrote that among the thousands of pregnant women he trained, nearly one in five reported feeling no pain in labor. Methods such as HypnoBirthing® encourage women to interpret the sensations of labor as *pressure* instead of pain and *surges* instead of contractions. Some women have simply said, "It was very strenuous work, but 'pain' is not the right word to express what I felt."

Here is how one mother portrayed her labor:

> Before I had my first baby, I was known as the member of my family with the lowest tolerance for pain. As my labor went on for four days, my doula helped me with every technique she could think of. At one point I rocked in a chair to relax, while looking out the hospital window at the river below. I started to daydream and think the view outside looked like Paris.
>
> My baby was born without my needing pain medication, and my memory after the birth was not that it was painful—which was a real surprise to my

family. My memory is that it was a beautiful experience I can tell my child about someday—and that I remember "going to Paris" in labor.

—Christina, 38, aesthetician, mother of five

## ⤳ SEXUALITY IN LABOR ⤳

Besides the fact that sex leads to pregnancy, what does lovemaking have to do with birth?

Some women describe having sexual feelings and orgasms during birth. This is because the hormones of labor and lovemaking are the same (oxytocin and the prostaglandins).

Sexual feelings are more likely to be reported by women giving birth in the privacy of their own homes, where they may be freer to actually incorporate lovemaking into their labors. Other women have described feeling sexual in labor without having sex.

Physical intimacy has excellent pain-relieving properties, and it speeds labor by increasing hormone levels. Even if you are not having a home birth, one of the best uses of your time at home in early labor is sensual or sexual touching, by yourself or with your partner.

Bringing sexuality into your labor can take many forms. Kissing or "making out" with your partner can be comforting and increase your sense of closeness. Breast or nipple stimulation helps speed up labor, and can be done by hand or mouth. While you are at home, breast stimulation should feel playful and fun, not like a clinical procedure. Stimulating your clitoris or having an orgasm can help increase your

## ᢙ SEXUALITY IN LABOR ᢙ

*(continued from previous page)*

uterine contractions; hands, mouth, or a vibrator on the outside of the body can be used for this purpose.

You can have intercourse or use penetration if your water hasn't broken; to prevent infection, do not insert anything into your vagina *after* your water breaks. Touching your cervix, or the presence of semen (which is rich in prostaglandins) on your cervix may help it open faster. And simply lying naked in skin contact with your partner will help increase oxytocin.

For more information about sexuality in labor, visit:

www.orgasmicbirth.com, Web site of the documentary film *Orgasmic Birth* made by Debra Pascali-Bonaro, an international leader in the doula movement;

http://susiebright.blogs.com, Web site of sexuality author Susie Bright, who wrote the essay "Egg Sex" about masturbation in labor;

www.unassistedchildbirth.com/sensual, Laura Shanley's Web site with a wealth of stories about sexuality in labor.

## YOUR FIRST LABOR IS AN ENDURANCE EVENT

The most unpredictable phase of childbirth is early labor with a first baby. Many women experience this phase in a gradual way, and it is hard to estimate exactly how long it will last. Contractions may start out twenty or thirty minutes apart, lasting less than thirty seconds each. Women can still talk normally or find that they only need to stop talking for a few seconds at a time during these early cramps.

The classic description of how labor evolves is that contractions become "longer, stronger, and closer together," and that's a fine explanation of exactly what happens. After increasing in strength every few hours, contractions will finally reach the point where they are about two to five minutes apart, lasting sixty to ninety seconds each (*active labor*). With each contraction, you'll need to stop talking for an entire minute now.

When contractions start out about twenty minutes apart, the length of labor will probably be average or longer. Less commonly for a first baby, a labor hits the ground running, with contractions coming five minutes apart from the beginning. This mother will probably have the advantage of a labor that is shorter than average. However, she'll have less time between contractions for a break, and she will need to mentally and physically adjust to being in strong labor right away.

Early labor with a first baby is likely to be at least ten or twenty hours, and may be as long as *two, three, or four entire days.* If you can imagine this in advance, you will be better able to handle the waiting involved before you ultimately reach active labor. Remember, early first labors that last several days are almost always completely normal, and they have the advantage of much longer breaks between contractions.

Contractions work by pulling on the lower portion of your womb (the *cervix*); in early labor this opens your cervix about halfway. During the rest of labor, your cervix will finish opening altogether, wide enough for your baby to pass through. Once active labor is reached, labor is more similar from woman to woman, and the baby will probably be born within the next five to ten hours.

## THE POWER OF ACTIVE LABOR

The beginning of active labor may be when you really wonder if you'll be able to handle the rest of the birth. Your labor will have shifted into higher gear several times before this point, and the beginning of active labor may be the most challenging thing you have ever physically experienced in life. (So far, that is.) You have finally reached the point where all your concentration is required. You will feel that you are being stretched to your limits, literally.

Your doula may coach you in techniques to help you welcome the feeling of contractions, or to distract you from them. As active labor continues, you will finally get used to this level of intensity. And then the intensity will increase again. Now you are being stretched to a new "limit." When labor shifts gears, it may take five or ten contractions to feel that you are on top of them again.

At a certain point, the intensity will probably reach a maximum level that will not become more painful as labor goes on. Contractions may come faster later, but not necessarily be more painful. It can be very helpful to have feedback at the point where "it won't get more painful than this" or "this is as hard as it will get." An experienced doula or nurse can help offer this judgment.

Late in labor a mother might be heard to say occasionally, "That contraction was an easy one." But if that particular contraction had occurred at the beginning of labor, she wouldn't have said that back then! Her capacity to handle the force of contractions has increased. Also, late in labor, some contractions *will* be easier than others—it's good to know they are not all going to occur at the maximum pain level.

Toward the end of labor, many women express normal feelings of uncertainty about how they will be able to continue. It is common to feel a mixture of determination, tearfulness, and doubt, and a wish to just be able to stop labor and go home.

You will find it incredible that labor gets stronger and stronger—and you do, too. The intense feeling of being overwhelmed, lacking control, or total surrender is the shortest part of labor. Welcome it as a normal part of the experience, one that signals you are nearly done!

A doula tells the following story:

> My client was in the middle of active labor. She turned to her partner and me, and said, "I don't know if I can do this, guys." We said we could see how tough it was, and she made it through that part. This happened three times. Finally she said, "That's it, I *really can't* do this anymore." Minutes later we found out her cervix was fully open and it was time to push the baby out!
>
> What was interesting was that she only said "I can't" once. Until then she was saying, "I *don't know* if I can," which was different. By the time she wanted to quit, she was at the end. I've seen this happen to many women—they say "I can't" just once, and then they have the baby.

Fathers and loved ones will have their own experience of the most intense moments of labor. Hearing a woman cry out at the end of labor can be unnerving for everyone witnessing it. It's helpful to know in advance that you are likely to witness this. Just as it is the shortest part of labor for the birthing mother, it will be temporary for you, too. Tears may be shed by pregnant women and their loved ones alike during the final trying moments of labor.

Because of the intensity of birth, it is the day of our lives that is often remembered more vividly than any other day. Exquisite sensitivity is needed to care for and respond to the needs of a newborn. If labor were not so attention-getting, we might have our babies, put them on our desks, and go back to answering our voice mail. The magnitude of labor prepares us mentally to focus on our newborns. It also prepares us biologically: in response to the effort and pain of labor, women's bodies produce extremely high levels of *endorphins* (natural painkillers and mood-boosters). After the baby is born, these endorphins remain, helping the mother and infant to bond.

## "IT'S COMING!"

The end of labor, when it's time to push your baby out, is the awesome and precious moment when you are about to finally become a parent. Various techniques for doing so have been the subject of much discussion and debate.

The most widely practiced style of pushing in the United States involves the doctor, midwife, or nurse coaching the mother to hold her breath for ten full seconds, three or four times during each contraction, and to bear down as forcefully as she can. (This type of breath-holding while straining is known as the *Valsalva maneuver,* which was originally developed to test pressure in the ears, and later used to test heart function.)

During birth, the Valsalva maneuver lowers the amount of oxygen the mother breathes to a minimum, and this reduction in oxygen can negatively affect the baby's heart rate. The technique of forceful pushing was developed without research showing it was beneficial; even so, it has been used on and off since at least the 1930s and currently predominates in maternity care. As of 2008, twelve studies have found no medical benefit to this style of pushing.

(Scholars are not sure why obstetricians began favoring the Valsalva maneuver; it may have coincided with the use of drugs that made it harder to feel pushing sensations, along with the use of certain positions that tend to slow labor.)

A pushing technique that was developed as a more "natural" alternative to the Valsalva maneuver involves asking the mother to hold her breath and bear down or strain for a shorter amount of time that she chooses, usually about five seconds.

We'd like to shed light on another approach that has

received less attention and deserves a wider audience: the option of *pushing with no added force.* There actually is pushing involved with this approach, however the mother does not intentionally add to the bearing-down efforts her body makes on its own, nor does she hold back. Over the years, various birth advocates have come to the conclusion that this would be beneficial. (In particular, this view of pushing is one of the most important contributions made by the HypnoBirthing® method, founded by Marie Mongan in the late 1980s.)

Because the baby must pass through your vagina, which sits right next to your rectum, the sensation of pushing will in some ways resemble an extremely intense bowel movement. One of the best ways to prepare for pushing is to pay attention to the way your bowel movements work and feel during pregnancy.

When you are lying down in bed and then get up, is that sometimes followed by the urge to have a bowel movement? Gravity is one of the most basic forces involved in elimination, and noticing the effect of your position may give you a preview of how gravity will work in your favor during labor.

If it's typical for you to actively bear down during bowel movements, try using no added force whatsoever. Practice this every time you use the bathroom. Gravity works along with *peristalsis* (your body's automatic movement of matter through your digestive system), and with the nerves around your vagina and rectum known as *stretch receptors.* The pressure of stool moving down activates the stretch receptors to make you push automatically.

A similar action happens in labor, known as Ferguson's reflex. The baby's head moves down naturally and triggers automatic pushing, without added force being necessary. Allowing this to happen on its own is referred to as *laboring down the baby;* after the cervix has fully opened, it can take minutes or hours before it actually begins. This waiting time can be crucial for successfully pushing out the baby.

Although many caregivers instruct women to start pushing even if they do not yet feel the urge, this will be about as effective as if you try to push out a bowel movement that is too high up; your body is just not able to perform this action yet. And according to studies in *Nursing Research* and the *American Journal of Obstetrics and Gynecology,* pushing too soon is more likely to drain the mother of energy, cause fetal distress, and lead to the use of forceps or a cesarean section.

While practicing on the toilet, if you feel you must strain or you will not be able to have a bowel movement, take a break and wait until later in the day when the urge to push feels stronger. Because pregnancy can be a time of increased constipation, you may have the perfect opportunity to try this out!

Also notice that the urge to push can be stronger or weaker at different times in the course of the same bowel movement. During birth, your pushing urges will also vary in strength. Your body will direct you as to how much or how little effort is needed for each push.

Even though the intention of aggressive pushing in labor is to speed up the process, studies show it may have the *opposite* effect and take longer. Heavy straining may cause the front wall of the vagina to be pushed down ahead of the baby. In this situation, the vaginal tissues may become "bunched up" and actually block or slow the descent of the baby, as well as damage the area where the vagina attaches to the bladder.

Bearing down forcefully during bowel movements, urination, and birth has been linked to problems such as hemorrhoids and bladder incontinence. In the case of childbirth, forceful pushing has even been associated with an increased risk of *prolapse,* or the bladder, uterus, or vagina coming out of the body. This may not become evident until later in life, but learning habits of gentle pushing now can help protect your organs from weakening for years to come.

As for the trend in pushing positions for birth, doctors most commonly ask women to assume the *lithotomy* position, or lying on one's back with knees bent and raised above the hips. This position is associated with more episiotomies and tears to the vagina. What position do mothers choose for pushing if they are not told what to do? In a study of 370 women published in the journal *Birth,* among mothers who were not told what position to use, only 5 percent *chose* to lie down!

(This is akin to asking, "What position do humans choose for having a bowel movement if they are not told what to do?")

On every continent of the world, the choice of women themselves has been to push in the upright positions. These include crouching, squatting, standing, kneeling, being on hands and knees, grasping something overhead, and even sitting on the toilet or a specially designed birth chair with a large hole in the seat.

Occasionally, pushing while lying on one's back might be the best position for that mother and baby. Although this is not common, a mother will be able to feel in her body if that position works better than others she has tried.

Your baby's task is to move from your belly and squeeze past your pubic bone, the bone behind the top of your pubic hair, in order to come out and be born. Though your baby's skull is firm, it is made of plates that are still movable so it can form a shape that will fit through your body, a process known as *molding* (sometimes resulting in a temporary "conehead" shape). Molding takes time. Once the right shape is formed, you will feel your baby's head suddenly slide down.

A mother tells the following story:

> At the end of labor, my doctor put his fingers inside my vagina and asked me to push his fingers out. He did this several times, and said I wasn't really doing it right yet. Finally he felt my baby move down and he said, "That's the right way to push!" But I

> know I was pushing exactly the same way I had been
> all along. My baby moved down because he found a
> way to fit through, not because I did anything differ-
> ently at all.
>
> —Leeza, 50, nonprofit worker, mother of one

A mild or moderate urge to bear down usually begins before the baby reaches its mother's pubic bone. However, *these
early sensations are not the same as real pushing.* These sensations
will build up until the baby begins to pass the pubic bone, at
which point the urge to push will become an overwhelming
force.

Providers who encourage pushing without added force, as
well as research published in October 2002 in the *American
Journal of Obstetrics & Gynecology,* have concluded that once the
baby naturally descends to the pubic bone, the "real" pushing
necessary to give birth almost always lasts less than a half hour,
even for first babies. On the other hand, the Valsalva maneuver takes an average of two hours of heavy straining without
an epidural, and an average of three hours with an epidural.

The first nine editions of *Williams Obstetrics* made no mention of coaching women to push. Then, in the 1950s, textbooks taught doctors to wait until the baby's head began to
show at the opening of the vagina before asking mothers to
push. But currently, providers encourage heavy pushing much
sooner, upon full opening of the cervix or the first several
urges to bear down. Usually though, it is still not the best time
to actively push! This is a time to let your body get used to the
increasing pressure of your baby moving toward your pelvic
floor, which is sometimes a startling sensation. Let your early
bearing-down urges simply be there, while neither resisting
them nor adding extra force to them.

Your baby's head and shoulders must first rotate in order
to fit through your pelvis. Intense pushing before this occurs

may only serve to "jam" your baby's head or shoulders above the brim of your pelvis. According to respected New Zealand midwife Jean Sutton, positions in which your knees are not pulled up toward your chest can give the baby more room to rotate into place. (E.g., standing or lying on your side with your knees below your hips.) Remember that *pushing too early,* or simply because the cervix has fully opened, can lead to difficulties.

Once your baby's head rotates, descends, and undergoes molding, it will settle in to pass your pubic bone. Finally, your baby is low enough to trigger your body's reflex of natural, active pushing! This wonderful moment is captured in the following story from Ms. Sutton, about her experience working in hospitals during an era when forceful pushing fell out of fashion in her locale:

> Thus, from 1951 to 1970, I saw hundreds of babies born. I had observed that mothers having a normal birth always said, breathlessly: "It's coming— never: I want to push." I never once saw a mother deliberately push her baby into the world—their uteri were quite capable of managing by themselves.

Most doctors and nurses are highly directive during pushing; that is, they coach the mother excitedly and loudly as to how to push. It has been said that the provider often has just as strong an urge to push as the mother. Although women do not naturally lie on their backs to push, hold their breath as long as possible, or bear down with extreme force, they are in a vulnerable state and it is hard for parents to regain control of the room once providers intensively begin coaching. Your body will give you many subtle cues about how and when to push, but it becomes harder to follow your body's messages when such strong directions are coming from others.

In order to have the experience of pushing with your body's own rhythm, it is necessary to remove instructions and coaching from others. Not only will this prevent the use of too much force, but an atmosphere of silence will best allow the mother to notice her own instincts.

### ASK YOUR DOCTOR NOW

If you'd like the option of pushing without added force, without lying down, or the option of silence, you will need to ask clearly for what you want. *Heavy coaching and placing women on their backs are some of the most tenacious routines in maternity care;* making other choices available takes strong advocacy from the parents.

Start these conversations during your prenatal appointments with your midwife or doctor. Will she or he support you in "laboring down" the baby for two hours or more? Has she ever seen a woman give birth in silence, without any instruction? If you want to stay off your back until the baby is completely out of your vagina, can she help with that? Which positions has she seen women use other than lying down for pushing? Write down your pushing preferences in your birth plan, which we'll be discussing further in chapter 11.

And in labor, discuss your wishes with the hospital staff *before* you get to the pushing stage, when intense coaching can take over the room quickly.

Pushing, delivering a baby, and holding a newborn in silence can be an awe-filled experience. The hormone oxytocin aids in pushing, as well as in creating feelings of love and protection in the mother toward her baby, and producing oxytocin is dependent on minimal disturbances by others in the room.

In 1957, one of the first studies on pushing was published under the title "The Normal Second Stage of Labor—A Plea for Reform in its Conduct." When women were allowed to push without straining, the research showed "better progress and greater ease [that] has to be witnessed to be believed," and less damage to the vagina; half a century later in 2006, the *New York Times* reported on a new study from the University of Texas Southwestern Medical Center that came to the same conclusion.

Remember, the approach of pushing without added force is something many U.S.-trained providers have never experienced, and it may not be possible to negotiate it in *exactly* the way it's been described in this chapter. There is no "right" way for you to push except for whichever one allows you to give birth to your baby safely. Spread the word about non-forceful pushing, and help make it an option again by knowing and informing others that it exists.

⌘ SEE THIS FILM ⌘

The film *Birth in the Squatting Position* is a little-known ten-minute video that has become a cult favorite among childbirth advocates. It shows mothers in a Brazilian hospital pushing in silence, without instruction, and is a highly moving portrayal of birth as we rarely see it today. If you want inspiration for what pushing can be like, the film is available on DVD from Cascade HealthCare Products, at 1-800-443-9942 or www.1cascade.com. If your midwife or doctor has a computer in her office, or if you have a laptop computer, bring this important video to your prenatal appointment and show it to your provider!

## IF YOU'VE GIVEN BIRTH BEFORE

Labor with a second or subsequent baby is different than labor with a first baby. If labor with a first baby is the hardest thing you'll ever do, labor with a second baby is not necessarily so.

Women having their second baby commonly bypass most of the early labor they experienced with their first. Within a few hours, you are likely to be in active labor. If you're pregnant and have already had a baby, take the time to imagine your upcoming labor being much shorter and slightly easier. You may be bracing yourself for a second labor that goes on for days if your first did so, but this is not what is likely to happen. Studies show women tend to expect their second labor to be like their first and overestimate how long or painful labor will be the second time.

You may have experienced medical procedures such as an epidural, Pitocin, or a cesarean with your first labor; you may be planning to avoid them this time, and curious about what labor will feel like without them. On the other hand, if you had medical interventions with your first baby, you may be expecting those procedures to be used again. However, they may not be entirely necessary, and your second birth may go more smoothly than a first labor that included interventions. You may be concerned that giving birth without an epidural or cesarean, and facing the effort of a normal labor, would involve more pain than you can handle.

If you are open to laboring without an epidural, review the descriptions of labor earlier in this chapter to prepare for the reality of what this will be like (minus early labor). Even if you plan to use an epidural for a second baby, labor may be short enough that there's not time for the drugs to make a big difference. If you are not open to laboring without an epidural for a second baby, enlist your doula to support your decision.

Discuss your first labor and any difficulties in your previous birth that you hope to avoid this time, and work together toward the birth that is best for you and your baby.

What about vaginal birth after a cesarean (VBAC)? Doctor support for VBAC increased in the 1990s and has decreased again since then, due to reports of the cesarean scar opening in labor, an unsafe event for the baby. In many cases, this was a result of commonly used drugs to induce or speed up birth. (According to sources including a 1999 report in the *American Journal of Obstetrics & Gynecology*, negative outcomes were more likely to be associated with the use of Cytotec [misoprostol]. Although widely and legally used, Cytotec carries a label from its manufacturer stating that it should not be used on pregnant women.) However, you may decline the use of drugs to stimulate labor.

The Cochrane Collaboration reports that VBAC involves overall levels of risk to the mother and baby that are lower than a repeat operation. In fact, a slight (non-dangerous) separation of the scar occurs in about 2 percent of mothers *before* birth, whether they are having a VBAC or another cesarean. Also, when a tear in the uterus does occur, the majority of the time a previous cesarean is not the cause. For more information, download the important booklet *What Every Pregnant Woman Needs to Know About Cesarean Section*, at www.childbirth connection.org.

Doulas play a vital role for mothers giving birth after a cesarean. First of all, the simple presence of a doula lowers the rate of cesareans. Secondly, doulas lower the use of epidurals and medications to stimulate labor, drugs that may increase the chances of a repeat cesarean. Finally, giving birth after a cesarean involves restoring your confidence that you can do it. (Yes, you can!)

According to cesarean expert Dr. Bruce Flamm, VBAC mothers have the same chance of achieving a vaginal birth as a woman who has never had surgery. Doulas help by discussing your emotions with you ahead of time, and supplying you with their faith and encouragement through every moment of labor; a Canadian study of thirteen hundred women showed that mothers with higher motivation for a VBAC were much more likely to achieve one.

# 4

# DRUGS, LAMAZE, AND BEYOND

In the midst of childbirth, how will you know whether to ask for pain medicine? Many women wonder about drugs. In truth, mothers in labor almost always know the answer to this question themselves.

If a woman asks, "Should I use drugs now?" her loved ones or doula can respond by saying, "What do you think?" If she replies, "Well, I'm not sure," that is not a yes. If she knows she is ready to request drugs, a mother normally will say clearly, "Yes, I am sure." A woman in labor is capable of making these decisions for herself; the job of her supporters is to listen carefully and affirm what she asks for.

A mother who is not sure she is ready for drugs needs the support to keep going without them. (This is for a normal labor. It would be insensitive and inhumane to tell a woman with abnormal levels of labor pain: "Keep going! Everything is fine!") A mother who is certain she is ready for medication usually needs support for her choice, not persuasion to do otherwise.

During birth, it is common for doctors and nurses to suggest to a woman that she use pain medication. Usually this is for the straightforward purpose of pain relief, although occasionally it is to correct what is seen as a medical problem, such as muscle tension in the mother which might be preventing the baby's descent. Because labor is a vulnerable and highly suggestible time, women who wish to avoid drugs find that these offers discourage them from their goal.

On the other hand, for women who plan to use drugs, offers from hospital staff may help them feel reassured they will not be denied. *The staff does not know whether you want to be offered drugs or you wish to have no offers; you need to clearly tell them.* This may save you hours of feeling unsupported or even undermined by a well-meaning nurse or doctor.

All women can get through a normal labor. This includes you. In order for this to happen, a woman needs feedback about what *is* normal. Doulas can help reflect whether labor pain is at a normal level and reassure you that yes, "You are having a good, normal labor. This is what normal labor looks like."

Whether you plan to use drugs or not, you can draw courage from the fact that women everywhere have the strength to give birth. While you're pregnant, do prepare for possible unexpected events in labor; but then return your focus to the likelihood that you and your baby will be fine, your body was smart enough to grow a baby and is smart enough to give birth, and you can do it.

## WHEN IS LABOR PAIN ABNORMAL?

When is the pain of labor outside the range of normal?

"Natural" contractions are most painful when a woman lies on her back. Even though these contractions are more painful, they are *less* effective at opening the cervix. If rest is needed, use a side-lying position to avoid maximum pain. Hospital staff often listen to the baby's heartbeat by instructing a woman to lie back, sometimes for long periods. However, you can request other positions for this, such as sitting or standing.

In cases where the drug Pitocin is used, there is a greater chance that labor pain will increase beyond what a woman can handle. However, the use of Pitocin does not always mean that an epidural will be required; if your plan was to avoid an epidural, be aware that you may still be able to do so. (See the section "How to Have a Great Pitocin Experience" in chapter 8.)

When it is time to push the baby out, women often feel relief. (Even so, the normal sensation of the baby emerging has been called "the ring of fire," because of the intense stretching of the opening of the vagina; this sensation only lasts a few minutes.) On rare occasions the pain of pushing may be worse than labor, and it is not too late to get an epidural for pain control even at this stage, if needed.

A stabbing pain in the abdomen that does not disappear between contractions is very uncommon, but can be a sign of an emergency with the placenta or uterus; bleeding heavier than a menstrual period can be another abnormal sign. If you experience either (or both) of these symptoms, notify your doctor or midwife immediately.

High stress and excess adrenaline in labor may cause

the lower portion of the uterus to close rather than open. Contractions may slow down in this situation, or they may continue with increased pain. If a birthing woman feels very fearful of the pain of labor, if she feels unsafe, or if support and guidance are not available to her, it is logical that body tension and doubts will increase, and the pain may indeed become unmanageable. Without a doula, this scenario can be common; the presence of a doula or another person experienced in normal birth can help lower the anxiety that leads to more pain.

## ᢒᔈ BACK LABOR: THE GOOD NEWS ᔔᢙ

In the past couple of decades, awareness has increased about *back labor,* or excessive pain felt in the lower back in labor. For years, back labor was believed to be caused by the baby being in a *posterior* position, meaning the baby's back is against the mother's back. This is not the best position for the baby to fit through the mother's pelvis, although it can be done; the ideal position is *anterior,* with the baby's back toward the mother's front.

Back labor is more painful than regular labor, and mothers and their providers have come to feel some dread about the possibility it will occur. However, groundbreaking research from Dr. Ellice Lieberman of Harvard Medical School in 2005 sheds new hope on this vexing situation. Lieberman's study involving over fifteen hundred mothers used ultrasound to determine the baby's position four times during each woman's labor.

What she found is that many babies change position all through labor. A posterior or anterior position at the beginning of labor does not predict the baby will stay that way until the end of labor. It may be that changes in the baby's position and even back labor are a normal part of many births, and can be viewed as temporary challenges that are likely to resolve later in labor.

Of course, back labor still hurts. The point here is to stay optimistic that labor is not "doomed" if it occurs. The best techniques to relieve the pain of back labor are for the mother to use forward-leaning positions, such as being on hands and knees, and for support people to press firmly against the mother's lower back, sometimes for hours.

Epidurals for back labor have their pros and cons; the extra back pain sometimes makes them more necessary. However, Lieberman's study found that with an epidural the baby's position was somewhat more likely to remain posterior and lead to a cesarean. To maximize chances of a baby rotating to the anterior with an epidural, use a "walking" epidural and continue changing the mother's position. (See the following section.)

In a few cases, back pain is not really *back labor*, it is a *back injury* that the mother had before or during pregnancy. If you feel excessive back pain in pregnancy, get it treated by a physical therapist, massage therapist, or chiropractor, so it will be less likely to flare up and cause problems in labor.

## "WALKING" EPIDURALS? YES!

If, in labor, you decide to say yes to drugs, you should know the good news about so-called "walking" epidurals. We spoke with anesthesiologist Dr. William Camann, a fan of doulas and coauthor of the book *Easy Labor,* who explains that these are simply lower doses of regular epidurals that can allow you to move around more than you would expect (and possibly, although not usually, literally walk).

For those who are already planning to get an epidural, this is by far your best choice. If you are planning not to get an epidural but find that you must, you'll be glad to know this isn't your mother's epidural. The amount of medication may be as little as one-tenth of the amount used in epidurals a generation ago.

When a low-dose epidural is used, pain relief is delivered, but there is less numbness and more of an ability to change positions. Staying active and upright may be the most important thing you can do to help labor unfold smoothly: contractions are stronger and there may be less need for Pitocin or a cesarean, the baby's head may turn more easily into the best position for birth, pushing is more effective when you are upright, and you may feel more psychologically in control than when you're lying down. With lighter epidurals, research shows that forceps and vacuums are used less often for delivery.

Though low-dose epidurals are now available in most hospitals, hospital staff often do not assist mothers in continuing to stay active and changing positions, or staff may outright discourage mothers from moving around. Even some doulas have been doubtful that there are benefits to a "walking" epidural, but we hope to reveal the well-kept secret that *you do* have more options with a lighter epidural.

While a low-dose epidural allows for more mobility than a high-dose epidural, individual results will vary, and a mother may still feel as though she is lacking some control over her movements. For safety, she should be assisted by hospital staff or her loved ones in taking on active positions. The good news is that a tremendous amount of mobility may still be available to her.

It is possible that you may be able to squat, kneel, sit on a birthing ball or rocking chair, get to the toilet rather than have a catheter or bedpan, or be on your hands and knees with a low-dose epidural. You may not need any direct assistance from others to assume these positions, although your helpers should stay next to you in case you feel that you cannot steady yourself.

In a 2006 study from the University Hospital Nice, France, published in the *International Journal of Obstetric Anesthesia,* mothers who received a very low-dose epidural were able to walk safely without falling or stumbling. (The medication used was 0.0625 percent bupivacaine, a lower amount of the standard drug used in nearly all epidurals.)

Even though position changes may be safe with a low-dose epidural, hospital staff usually assume that women will not actually wish to stay active, even with a "walking" epidural. With most epidurals, hospital staff commonly encourage women to go to sleep. They often assume this is what a mother wants with a lighter epidural, too.

Squatting is especially helpful when it is time to push the baby out. This position is probably the most effective one available for pushing, because it opens your pelvis to its widest dimension and uses the forces of gravity to bring your baby down and out of your body. However, most doctors are trained to place women on their backs and will frequently coach mothers to "push your baby out toward the ceiling!" (This is one of the strangest things often heard in labor and delivery.) A low-dose epidural is more likely than a high-dose epidural to allow you to squat to push your baby out.

## ⤳ ASK YOUR DOCTOR NOW ⤳

If you would like the option to squat or change positions with an epidural, you'll need to clearly let your providers know. Start having these conversations with your doctor or midwife at your prenatal appointments. If getting out of bed with an epidural is not permitted at your hospital, ask what other positions they feel would be safe for you to use.

In labor, remind the hospital staff that it's your goal to change positions with an epidural, and ask for their encouragement and physical assistance to do so.

So how do you know if you're getting a "walking" epidural? In fact, the standard epidural at many hospitals would actually qualify. Many hospitals now start with a lower dose of drugs, and then give you the option of increasing the drugs throughout labor. The more the drugs are increased, the less ability you'll have to move around.

Most women report that the lower dose meets their needs well, but occasionally epidurals seem as though they're not working. Before going to a higher dose of drugs, try changing positions first. Epidurals work with gravity, and if you're lying on your left side, your right side may feel as though it's not getting pain relief; in this case, simply turn to lie on your right, and give it fifteen to thirty minutes to work.

As you get near the end of labor, the epidural may seem to be wearing off, but it is not. What is actually happening is that contractions are getting stronger. The increasing sensations are usually manageable, and if you can hold off from going up on the drugs, you will be more able to achieve upright positions for pushing.

I asked for a low-dose epidural, and I changed positions at least ten times after I got it, without physical help from anyone. During pushing, my doctor
ran in and out of the room several times because
another woman was in labor. Each time she came in
and saw me squatting she said, "Oh, that looks like
your favorite position. Fine!" and ran out again. I
could tell clearly which positions felt "right" and
helped move my baby down, and which positions
didn't, and I kept changing in response to this.

—Serena, 30, accountant, mother of two

Perhaps the main reason "walking" epidurals have been
viewed with doubt is that most hospital staff and mothers have
*simply never tried* to use them to stay mobile. The term "walking" epidural has caused confusion, but it's not so important
that an epidural be called this, or that walking happens. What
matters is that it be given at a low dose, and active positions
continue to be safely used.

If you get an epidural, talk with the anesthesiologist about
how to keep the dose low. He or she may choose to deliver the
drugs more slowly through the tube, use a different combination of drugs, start with a lower dose, or simply advise you not
to keep raising the level of drugs throughout labor. He might
also decide to use an alternate procedure known as the *com-
bined spinal epidural.* Each doctor's approach will vary, so communicate and work cooperatively with your anesthesiologist
to achieve the goal you want.

"Walking" epidurals are not pure magic; they can have all
the same side effects as high-dose epidurals, including lowering
the mother's blood pressure and affecting the baby's heart rate.
But they offer benefits that surpass those of traditional epidurals. Also, staying upright may minimize the side effects of an
epidural, including low blood pressure, and might make all the
difference between a positive and negative birth experience.

Studies show that most women report greater satisfaction with a lighter epidural. However, in some situations a higher dose truly is needed in order to provide the appropriate pain control. Even in these cases, you can usually still assume more positions than only lying down. You will need physical assistance from others, but you'll probably be able to sit completely upright in bed, with your back against the headboard or your legs over the side of the bed, or you may be able to get onto your hands and knees with the support of a stack of pillows under your torso, for example.

In 2007, the scientific journal *Nature* reported that doctors at Massachusetts General Hospital are developing a new type of anesthesia that may be able to *completely* separate pain relief from motor functions. This could someday make walking in labor a possibility for any mother with an epidural. As of this writing, the drug is being tested on rats and sheep before moving on to human trials. Stay tuned.

## WHETHER TO LEARN A "METHOD"

Is it necessary to learn specific techniques ahead of time, or practice your breathing, or otherwise train for childbirth? Truthfully, no. Birthing classes are not mandatory, either.

You already know how to perform the actions that can be some of the most useful in labor: get out of bed, walk around, touch your loved ones, and take really long showers as a form of pain relief at the hospital, where they never run out of hot water. We'll talk more later about how to make the most of these techniques, but training is not required.

Childbirth classes serve a useful social function, introducing you to other expectant parents. Watching birth films in class and discussing what happens in labor can help the upcoming event feel more real. According to Childbirth Connection, approximately 95 percent of birth classes are affiliated with hospitals or clinics; these are sometimes thought of by childbirth advocates as "obedience classes," because they may teach you to be more of a passive patient than an active, informed consumer.

Classes that are more commonly offered outside of hospitals, and that can help you be more empowered during birth, include:

- Active Birth (primarily U.K.), which emphasizes the importance of upright positions rather than lying down; www.activebirthcentre.com
- ALACE classes (primarily U.S. and Canada), which promote "woman-centered" birth and following the woman's instincts; www.alace.org
- Birthing From Within (U.S. and international), an approach based in psychological exercises and art therapy; www.birthingfromwithin.com
- The Bradley Method® (primarily U.S. and Canada), an intensive twelve-week series that encourages you to take responsibility for your birth; www.bradleybirth .com
- HypnoBirthing® (U.S. and international), which teaches simple methods of relaxation through self-hypnosis for those who wish to have techniques to practice ahead of time; www.hypnobirthing.com

If you don't learn a "method" before labor, do not worry that you will be unprepared to cope. It is not even required that you feel 100 percent confident in order to give birth. Your body knows how to labor whether or not you have studied techniques; what will be most useful to you are the things that comfort you in everyday life, and minute-by-minute support from your loved ones and doula. (In recent years, even the Lamaze organization greatly relaxed its focus on the strict breathing techniques that made it famous.)

---

There are also a variety of other ways you can get ready to welcome your baby, if you're contemplating how to go about it. Here are some of our favorites:

### Yoga, Pilates, and Meditation

These practices encourage you to breathe deeply while holding an intense stretch or position for a full minute or longer. If you've tried these techniques, deep breathing for relaxation will come to you more easily in labor (which also involves a muscle, your uterus, holding an intense position for a full minute).

### Massage Therapy

Yes, this is actually a form of childbirth preparation. According to pilot studies from the Touch Research Institute at the University of Miami, if you are able to go to a massage therapist a half-dozen times while pregnant, the relaxation effects can carry over to help you have an easier labor. We can't think of a better justification for getting a massage.

---

### TO FIND
### ⤳ A MASSAGE THERAPIST ⤳

You can ask if massage is offered at your gym, hair salon, or local hotel. Otherwise, in the U.S., contact the American Massage Therapy Association at www.amtamassage.org or Associated Bodywork & Massage Professionals at www.massagetherapy.com/find.

## Vaginal Exercises

Exercises known as *Kegels* help your pelvic muscles to be in better condition, which may help your baby fit more easily through your body as he is born, and your vagina may recover more quickly after birth. Simply tense the muscles around your vagina as if stopping a flow of urine and then release. (However, do not regularly do Kegels with a full bladder.) After releasing, it's optional to bear down *lightly,* not forcefully. Look for a time to do at least thirty per day for eight weeks, for example while talking on the phone. Kegels can also increase your ability to have an orgasm.

## Working Out at the Gym

Actually, *any* kind of cardio exercise or strength training can help strengthen your pelvic muscles. Toward the end of pregnancy, swimming is a great option when other kinds of vigorous exercise feel unmanageable. Swimming helps develop your ability to breathe deeply, usually feels good to an aching back, and might even help turn a baby who is in a breech position.

## Perineal Massage

You or your partner can gently massage the outside and inside of your vagina with plain vegetable oil or a lubricant like K-Y Jelly in whatever way feels good to you. If you try this, have fun with it; this is not a medical procedure! Think of this as a treat for a part of your body that'll be working hard during the upcoming big event. The most current studies show this might reduce chances of vaginal tissues tearing during birth.

## USING BELLY DANCE FOR BIRTH

Helping Jennifer Wright through labor in the delivery room of a Missouri birthing center in early 2007 were her doctor, her husband—and her belly-dance instructor.

With the teacher, DeeDee Farris-Folkerts, by her side reminding her of the moves, Ms. Wright stood holding her husband while doing the hip circles and pelvic rotations characteristic of the ancient Arabian dance. She had readied a compact disc with classic Egyptian music, but didn't have a chance to play it before her daughter, Aubrey, emerged.

"I danced my way through labor," says Ms. Wright, the mother of three, who had been given painkillers and labor-inducing medication during her oldest child's birth and wanted a natural alternative. Her husband, Joe Walls, says he learned that belly dancing "is more than just entertainment. It has a much higher purpose."

These days, alternative techniques to ease labor run the gamut from hypnotherapy to "water births" in a large bathtub. But some women disillusioned with routine use of medical interventions during labor are turning to an unusual solution—belly dancing. They're restoring the titillating dance of seduction—frequent entertainment fare in nightclubs and Middle Eastern restaurants—to what they say were its origins in childbirth, while enhancing maternity wards with swirling motions and mesmerizing music.

Expectant mothers can choose from an increasing array of prenatal belly-dancing classes and educational materials. The first instructional prenatal belly-dance DVD in the U.S. was released in 2006, with a pregnant dancer named Naia leading the class.

"Most of the women who come to me have given birth

before and they want something different," says Ms. Farris-Folkerts, who typically has three to eight pregnant students in her belly-dance courses, and is also a doula.

The belly dance arrived in the U.S. in the 1890s, according to belly-dance lore, when impresario Sol Bloom brought an "Algerian" village to the Chicago World's Fair and introduced the dancer Little Egypt, who cavorted to improvised snake-charmer music. Incorporating elements of striptease and so-called hootchie-cootchie dancing, the belly dance gained its come-hither reputation.

British anthropologist Sheila Kitzinger says belly dancing originated as a ritual of childbirth as well as seduction. Among Bedouin Arabs, she says, girls are taught a pelvic dance during puberty to celebrate their budding sexuality and prepare for the physical marathon of childbirth.

Some belly-dance movements mirror those of labor. The idea is that the pelvic gyrations help disperse the pain of contractions, orient the fetus, and propel the baby into the world. In early labor, when contractions are relatively mild, the expectant mother may find comfort in dancing slowly and hypnotically, using hip circles, crescents, and figure eights. As labor gets more intense, the movements may progress to a rapid rocking of the pelvis from side to side—a technique known as the shimmy—to help position the baby correctly and relax the pelvic floor. In the final phase of pushing, a full body undulation known as the camel roll can help the baby move into the birth canal.

A New York dancer who calls herself Morocco popularized the link between dancing and childbirth in the late 1960s with a firsthand account of a birth and dance ritual near Casablanca. Two decades later, a troupe called the Goddess Dancing was formed in greater Boston to celebrate the roots of belly dancing and teach classes to pregnant women and others.

Chris Willow-Schomaker taught herself to belly dance

from a video before her second son was born at home. When contractions started coming quickly, she played dance music and did full circles and swings moving her whole belly. "Then I would raise my hands high and tell the baby, 'Down, baby, down, come on down, baby.'" A few hours later, Silas was born.

"The movements that women make when they're belly dancing are the same movements that I am trying to get them to make to bring the baby down," says her doctor, Elizabeth Allemann.

One difference between those who belly dance onstage and in delivery rooms is belly size. When Stefanie Masters teaches her prenatal class at a maternity clothing store in Wisconsin, she waives her usual dress code for belly-dance students, which calls for exposed bellies. "Thirty to seventy pounds in pregnancy can be pretty emotionally traumatic," she says. "I want the women to feel good about themselves and enjoy the process." Her pregnant pupils do wear hip belts, with tiny dangling coins that "make a beautiful jingly sound when your hips move."

Susan Swearingen says she was transformed after taking her first class from Ms. Masters last year. "My mood, my anxiety lifted," she says. "It helped my posture and my confidence. I felt beautiful when I was dancing."

Ms. Swearingen says she practiced "pretty hard-core belly dancing" in early labor at home. Then at the hospital, she embarked on shimmies, camel rolls, and large pelvic circles, sometimes holding hands with her husband. At one point, she says, the medical log on a computer screen in her hospital room read, "Dancing with husband."

Madeline McNeely "belly danced" on all fours when she went into labor at home. "I had to crawl from the bedroom, across the apartment, down the stairs, and into the car because I couldn't stand up," says the leadership consultant.

"As I was crawling, I was moving my hips, doing the hip circles. That circle feeling made a huge difference."

Cathy Moore, a midwife at Brigham and Women's Hospital in Boston who also performs with the Goddess Dancing group, is slowly introducing belly-dance techniques to some patients and birth specialists. The vanity plate on her Volkswagen Jetta reads: BELLY.

At a 2007 childbirth conference outside Boston, giggling, suburban nurses struggled to mimic Ms. Moore's rapid-fire body shakes. "Do you feel all those muscles loosening?" called out Ms. Moore, sporting a belly-dance costume of hip-hugging skirt and bejeweled halter top. "Can you see how this helps labor?"

Ms. Moore says she has to tread carefully at the Brigham because for some expectant moms, belly dancing remains outside the medical mainstream. She also notes that certain movements should be avoided: sharp hip drops and pops, and anything up on the toes. James Greenberg, the hospital's vice chairman of the department of obstetrics and gynecology, says he's not sure if belly dancing offers proven benefits. "But there's certainly no scientific reason to think it's bad, so if it makes you feel good, and it's safe, do it."

## OTHER PREPARATIONS TO MAKE

We encourage you to use your prenatal visits with your provider to start conversations about birthing issues that are important to you. This is one of the most important ways in which you can prepare for birth. (You will notice sections in this book titled "Ask Your Doctor Now," which you can use as starting points for these talks.)

Give your doctor or midwife time to respond thoroughly to your questions; you may be surprised or reassured by her answers. If you sense the topic is controversial, ask your provider to show you research on it the next time you meet. In the meantime, do your own research on the Cochrane Collaboration database at www.cochrane.org, or ask your doula to help you locate it, and bring it with you for further discussion with your provider. There will be little or no time for these conversations in labor, so make the most of your prenatal appointments in this way.

Every time a patient asks her provider to discuss issues that are important to her, it benefits her and other mothers. These may be the only times in which caregivers learn what is truly on the minds of their patients. Doctors usually leave explanations of childbirth to the teachers of birth classes, but in doing so, pregnant women miss out on having a dialogue directly with the person responsible for patients' care. Also the beliefs and practices of doctors may not be the same as what is taught by childbirth teachers. Don't skip the chance to have these talks with your provider.

---

Finally, watch other women breastfeed. While you're pregnant, start going to meetings for mothers who are already breastfeeding, such as the international organization La Leche League (www.lalecheleague.org) or a postpartum support group at your hospital. A breastfeeding class for pregnant women may also be helpful, but you will learn even more at a group where mothers bring their babies because *you'll see how* they breastfeed. Also you will meet experienced mothers whom you can call when you're back home with your baby, if and when you need help with breastfeeding. If you have friends who are nursing and you feel comfortable, ask them to show you how they breastfeed and to talk with you about what helped them succeed.

> I'm seventeen and I had twins. In the hospital after I gave birth, my doula was helping me and my

husband learn how breastfeeding works. When my friends came to visit that day, some of them said, "We breastfed and we're going to make sure you do." Knowing they did it at my age helped give me confidence that I could, too.

—Mavis, 17, student, mother of two

# 5

# FIND YOUR DOULA!

Finding a doula is a bit like finding a good plumber or a piano teacher; to learn who is available, you'll simply need to start making phone calls. Most doulas work for themselves, often from home, and to reach them you will be calling them directly. About 20 percent of doulas work for a hospital or a community program, which means that you will contact the program first to be referred to a doula.

You can start your search for a doula at any time during your pregnancy. We recommend meeting labor assistants near the end of your second trimester, when you are about six months pregnant, so you'll have time to look for and interview them in a relaxed manner. This is also when you may be taking childbirth classes, and it's a good time to talk with your doula about what you are learning. But if you find yourself at the end of your pregnancy without a doula, it is not too late to look for one.

Begin by asking friends, as well as your doctor or midwife, if they can refer you to doulas they have worked with. You might need to make several calls to find a doula who has availability for the month of your due date, because each doula can only take on a limited number of clients per month. If the first person you contact is not available, ask her for names of other doulas. Sometimes it takes persistence, but it is well worth it for you to keep looking.

In addition to word of mouth, you can contact the national and international doula organizations (listed on the next page). These organizations certify or offer membership to doulas and maintain lists of their members for referrals to the general public. You can call these groups, or go right to their Web sites to find names of doulas. You can also search the Internet to find doulas in your area. Use a search engine such as Google and type in "doula," along with the name of your city, state, province, or country.

## Doula Groups—U.S. and Canada

### United States

Association of Labor Assistants
and Childbirth Educators
www.alace.org
888-22-ALACE

Childbirth and Postpartum
Professional Association
www.cappa.net
888-MY-CAPPA

DONA International
www.dona.org
888-788-DONA

### Canada

Association of Labor Assistants
and Childbirth Educators
www.alace.org
888-22-ALACE

CAPPA Canada
www.cappacanada.ca
866-CDN-BIRTH

DONA International
www.dona.org
888-788-DONA

## Doula Groups—Outside North America

### Australia

Find A Doula
www.findadoula.com.au

### Austria

Doulas in Austria
www.doula.at

### Belgium

L'Association Francophone des
Doulas de Belgique
www.doulas.be

### Brazil

Doulas do Brasil
www.doulas.com.br

### Czech Republic

Czech Doula Association
www.duly.cz

### France

Doulas de France
www.doulas.info

### Germany

Wir Doulas in Deutschland
www.doula-info.de

### Hungary

Association of Hungarian
Doulas
www.module.hu

**Ireland**

Doula Ireland
www.doulaireland.com

**Israel**

www.doula.co.il

www.dulot.co.il

**Netherlands**

www.doula.nl

**Portugal**

Doulas de Portugal
www.doulasdeportugal.org

**South Africa**

South African Doula Database
http://doulas.co.za

**Spain**

www.doulas.es

**Switzerland**

www.doula.ch

**United Kingdom**

Doula UK
http://doula.org.uk

## COMMUNITY DOULAS

Although most doulas are hired on a private basis by their pregnant clients, community doula programs have also been developed by some nonprofit organizations and agencies.

"Community-based doulas" are recruited from the populations they serve, providing peer support for mothers with increased social needs, including teenage, low-income, and minority mothers. The most well-known of the community-based programs is the Doula Project of the Chicago Health Connection (CHC), begun in 1996 with a focus on serving teen mothers. CHC created a program to duplicate its work, and has done so with approximately thirty-four doula programs in Arizona, Colorado, Georgia, Illinois, Indiana, Minnesota, New Mexico, and Washington. CHC has also sponsored conferences for community-based doulas from around the United States. For information on their work, contact:

Chicago Health Connection
www.chicagohealthconnection.org
312-243-4772

## SUPPORTING TEENS:
### ᏰᏰ A TALK WITH JANE FONDA ᏰᏰ

Jane Fonda, actor, philanthropist, activist, and mother, is founder and chairperson of the Georgia Campaign for Adolescent Pregnancy Prevention, or G-CAPP, a nonprofit organization. G-CAPP's doula program for teen mothers was launched in 2002 and has already had an impact—higher breastfeeding rates among the doula-supported young mothers, more time before a subsequent pregnancy, fewer premature and low-birth-weight babies and fewer C-sections and epidurals. Ms. Fonda envisions the doula program taking root throughout the U.S. In a March 2008 interview, we spoke to Ms. Fonda about how she became such a powerful advocate for doulas:

"About ten years ago, the Clinton administration was in the process of launching what has become a national campaign to prevent teen pregnancies. There was a roomful of people, including Hillary and about thirty to thirty-five others, all of whom were involved in adolescent pregnancy prevention.

"In there was a man named Irving Harris—I did not know him. He gave me his card and I gave him mine. And in the course of the next year or so he would send me letters and speeches that he'd made and articles that he'd written, and most of them had to do with the doula project.

"He was the one that helped me see the relationship between good early parenting and bonding with the child and the later reduction in adolescent pregnancies.

"I had heard of a doula but didn't really know what a doula was. I knew that we have a hospital here that has doulas, and usually it's middle-class girls that get them and they come in at the time of birth. But this was different.

"Eventually, I went to Chicago with the CEO of G-CAPP to see what this was all about. We were really impressed. Now, the way that the program works is that you identify women in the community of the same ethnicity as the girls that they are going to be paired with. So most of the doulas were African-American and Hispanic, a few Caucasian. Many of them were themselves adolescent parents, some of them had never worked before. Every community has leaders in it, indigenous leaders that go under the radar, who, with a little training, rise to the surface and become leaders.

### LEADERS FROM THE COMMUNITY

"So we identify these women, then train them intensively for four months, paying them while they're being trained. And the training is very interesting. Yes, they're being trained on prenatal care and postnatal care, and child development, but more than that we start off helping these women to deal with their own childbirth trauma. Many of them went through their own childbirth without support and with some difficulty. There was old stuff kind of stuck there that they had to work through before they could

## SUPPORTING TEENS:
### A TALK WITH JANE FONDA

*(continued from previous page)*

realize their full potential as doulas. So in some ways the training was profoundly transformational for the doulas.

"When they graduate, they are then paired with a supervisor and then they are matched up with the young girls who are pregnant. And again, the time leading up to the birth is not just making sure that these young girls get their prenatal care, but it's about bonding with these girls and it's important to understand that the population we are dealing with here is a population of young women who have never had a primary attachment.

"They've never had an adult really care about them. Try to understand what it's like: you're young, you're maybe fourteen years old, you have nobody with you, nobody helping you, and you enter this system which is a hospital, and you're in labor. It's utterly terrifying.

"These girls have an adult who they've bonded with, who they trust, and who has asked them to begin to think of this growing child as a human being, not just something that's making them feel uncomfortable and keeping them from going out with their friends. This is a future human being that they are going to be responsible for, and to begin to think about what their vision of the future is, and to write it, even write letters to this unborn child. For these girls it's a big deal. They haven't been taught to think in those ways.

"Just the notion of thinking about a future, in fact, can be foreign to them. It's very profound.

### BIRTH

"Then, the second part is when this young woman gives birth. I remember learning about how important a doula can be, when one of the leaders of the doula program, Dr. Marshall Klaus, came to my home. We were at the stage of trying to get partners and people involved in the doula project and we brought him in to speak to legislators. So we were all gathered in my apartment and he began to stroke my thigh and look into my eyes and he said, someone doing this while you are in labor, the touching and stroking of your arm or thigh, the looking into your eyes, what we have seen is that this reduces most of the problems and difficulty with labor—reduces the need for cesareans, the need for drugs and a host of other things. It allows the young mother to relax. Just the loving presence of someone and the effective touch—it just blew my mind because this was a doctor, he was an expert in this.

"So that's what the doula does, she is not a midwife, she is more of a coach who touches and countenances and gives emotional support and nurtures and when the baby is born, she encourages the mother to breastfeed.

"Now another thing people may not know— it seems counterintuitive—but these girls don't breastfeed.

"Their grandparents did and you'd think it's what they'd do—it's free and it's mother's milk and it's also very healthy for the child—but it's not considered cool.

## SUPPORTING TEENS: A TALK WITH JANE FONDA

*(continued from previous page)*

"So it's a big deal to get these young girls, mostly girls of color, to breastfeed.

"And it's hard to make that up, if you miss that window of opportunity, in terms of skin time and bonding, you know, you have to work extra hard to make up for it later.

### POSTPARTUM

"Then for four months after birth, the doulas go into the home and help the young mothers understand, for example, that it's normal that the baby is crying, that colic is normal, that it doesn't mean she's a bad mother. 'Look how smart your baby is, he knows your voice already. Look how his head follows your voice, look how he reaches out to grab your finger.' Suddenly the mother is helped to see her child not as a bundle of problems and poop, but, 'Hey, my child is smart, he knows me, I could be a good mother.'

"Those of us who've had kids know that this is the time we're most open, most sponge-like, most able to receive information, to learn, we want to learn. We want to be helped. And it's a tremendous teaching window of opportunity. And when women at this stage are made to feel they are empowered mothers, it changes everything: they don't want to leave their baby with a boyfriend, they stop doing drugs, they don't drink while they're breastfeeding, abuse goes down.

## LONG-TERM STRATEGY

"What the late Irving Harris believed and certainly what I believe, is if you did a longitudinal study, when these young children grow up they won't become teen parents or at least not in the numbers that we would have seen before because they have received that kind of bonding with a loving adult, with their parent, early on in life. And it's the lack of love; it's as basic as that, the lack of love and the lack of hope that kind of keeps these young people from protecting themselves if they are sexually active and avoiding risky behavior. So it's like a long-term primary pregnancy prevention strategy, I think. But it's also a secondary pregnancy prevention strategy. Because these mothers, when they see what it really takes to be a mother, they don't want to have another baby right away. That appears to be the case in Georgia—and that's the experience they've had in the Chicago Doula Project—that second pregnancies are greatly reduced. That's one of the main reasons we brought the program here.

## THE FUTURE

"My dream would be to embed this program in WIC [the program that delivers food and infant formula to poor women and children]. It's a natural fit: they have this population of at-risk girls who are pregnant and parenting. We've talked about the doula project to women who work in WIC offices and they cry, they say, 'We're just skimming the surface, if we could get this program, our work would be so much

## SUPPORTING TEENS:
## ᘓᓇ A TALK WITH JANE FONDA ᓇᘗ

*(continued from previous page)*

deeper.' So [with the new presidential adminis-
tration], one of my first jobs will be to go up
there and try to persuade them to look at
this."

## HOSPITAL AND SPECIALTY DOULAS

Other local and specialty doula programs exist nationally and
internationally. Some hospitals and birth centers run their
own doula programs and make their services available to any
woman birthing at their facilities, or to women with certain
needs, such as speaking another language. (The benefit of such
programs is that services may be available at no cost to the
woman; the downside is that hospital-based labor assistants
report feeling less effective at being an advocate for the mother,
due to also being a hospital employee.) A listing of such programs is being compiled by DONA International, along with
Ann Fulcher of the Doula Program at the University of
California, San Diego Medical Center. For more information
on finding a hospital-based doula program near you, go to
www.dona.org.

Doula programs and referral Web sites have also been developed to address the needs of various populations; some of
these resources are listed on the following page.

## African-American

International Center for
    Traditional Childbearing
    (U.S.A.)
Full Circle Doula program
http://blackmidwives.org
503-460-9324

African American Doula
    Directory (U.S.A.)
www.blackdoulas.com

## American Indian

American Indian Family Center
    (Minnesota, U.S.A.)
Turtle Women Community
    Doula Program
www.aifc.net
651-793-3803

## Christian

Christian Midwives
    International (U.S.A.)
Referrals to Christian midwives
    and doulas
www.christianmidwives.org

## Incarcerated

The Birth Attendants
    (Washington, U.S.A.)
www.birthattendants.org
The Birth Attendants,
    PO Box 12258, Olympia,
    WA 98508

Birth Companions (London,
    U.K.)
Doulas for women in detention
www.birthcompanions.org.uk
Birth Companions, PO Box
    56431, London SE3 7UZ

## Lesbian

Web site about lesbian and gay
    parenting (U.S.A.)
www.prideparenting.com
For doulas, click on
    "Reproduction," then click
    on "Links"

## Military

Operation Special Delivery
    (U.S.A.)
Doulas for women whose part-
    ners are deployed
www.operationspecialdelivery
    .com
888-MY-CAPPA

## Substance Abuse

The Believe Project (Boston,
    U.S.A.)
A program of the Birth Sisters
    at Boston Medical Center
www.bu.edu/obgyn/clinical/
    sisters.htm
617-414-5168

## DOULA SPECIALTY: ADOPTION AND SURROGACY

At the birth of a baby whose family is being formed through adoption or surrogacy, the pregnant mother as well as the adoptive parents have special vulnerabilities and needs, as do other family members who may be present. (With surrogacy, the parents who will be raising the baby are commonly referred to as the "intended parents.") A number of doulas are available to assist at adoptive births, and they can be helpful to each of the parties involved. Some adoption agencies encourage the use of doulas, which may be how you learned about them.

As part of our research for this section, we spoke with Kate MacLellan, a doula who was herself adopted, who adopted and breastfed her first two children, and birthed her third child. Kate lives in Canada, specializing in attending births as a doula for mothers who are placing their babies for adoption, and she is a trainer for the adoption certification program offered by the doula organization CAPPA.

Each person and family experiencing adoption or surrogacy will have their own different wishes about what will happen at the baby's birth. The purpose of this section is to introduce some of the options available, even though you might not use all of them at your birth.

### Birth Mothers

As with any birth, the primary focus of the doula at an adoptive or surrogate birth will be on the mother in labor. The needs of the pregnant woman's extended family, as well as the intended or adoptive parents, will also be strong; however their needs will not necessarily be the same as those of family members at a traditional birth.

Some doulas have observed that ideally, *two* doulas should be available at an adoptive birth, one for the birth mother and one for the adoptive parents. This might be an option, but if not, one labor assistant may be able to help with the needs of the various parties.

Birth mothers often choose not to participate in regular childbirth classes, where their plans for their baby would be different than those of the traditional couples present. A doula can give the birth mother private childbirth classes or help find a teacher for this. In some cases, the birth father will also be present at the birth, and he can participate in meetings with the doula as well. Or the birth father may not be present, and the birth mother may choose another family member as her support person, such as her own mother.

With adoption and surrogacy, the birth mother's extended family may or may not support her decision to place her baby with another family. For example, if the grandmother will be present at the birth, but does not support the adoption, it can be helpful for the doula to meet alone with the birth mom, in order to fully focus on her needs and wishes. At a later time, the grandmother can join in meetings with the doula, so that all may prepare together for what to expect during birth.

### Adoptive and Intended Parents

If the intended or adoptive parents will be present at the birth, they too will be in need of information about childbirth. The doula may be able to provide this. It can be helpful for the labor assistant to meet with the adoptive parents separately from the birth mother, with the permission of all parties. Confidentiality on the part of the doula is important in this situation, so that birth parents as well as adoptive parents can freely express their emotions and needs.

Adoptive or intended mothers may plan to breastfeed their new babies, even if they have never given birth before. A doula with breastfeeding experience may be able to help with this. In order to build a supply of milk, treatment is started as early as six months before the baby's birth. A breast pump is used daily, and hormones may or may not also be taken to stimulate the production of milk. It is possible the adoptive mom may be able to produce a full milk supply for the baby's needs. For more information, visit the Web site of adoptive breastfeeding expert Lenore Goldfarb, at http://asklenore .info.

### Labor and Delivery

With surrogacy, there is usually more contact prenatally between the birth mother and the intended parents than with adoption, and the intended parents are commonly present at the baby's birth.

With adoption, the birth mother may feel comfortable inviting the adoptive parents to the birth, or she may choose not to, due to her own needs for privacy, or if she is still undecided about placing the baby for adoption. Some adoptive parents are enthusiastic about being present at the birth, while others choose not to, because of the chance the baby might not ultimately go home with them. In either case, a doula can support the laboring woman.

Adoptive or intended parents may experience feelings of amazement and gratitude while watching the birth, as well as jealousy or pain if they experienced their own fertility or reproductive health problems.

If the adoptive parents are not in the delivery room, the birth mother may wish to have them stay in the waiting room, so they can care for the baby right after the birth. Or, rather than having them wait in the hospital, the birth mother may decide to call the adoptive parents immediately after the birth to come to the hospital.

Hospitals are becoming more sensitive about adoption and surrogacy; however, your hospital's policies may not easily accommodate your family. For example, some hospitals are strict about limiting the number of support people present in the birthing room to two. This means that if the birth father, grandmother, one or two doulas, and the surrogate or adoptive parents wish to attend the birth, they may not all be allowed.

Be sure to inquire if there is a limit at your hospital, and if so, ask if an exception can be made to include the support people of the birth mother's choosing. If an exception is made, ask that the hospital put the arrangements into writing ahead of time. The birth mom is not obligated to have a large crowd, but she should bring the number of people that is best for *her*.

### Postpartum

When the baby is born, the birth mother will choose what amount of contact she would like with the baby. She can be the first to hold the baby, or she can ask the intended or adoptive parents to be the first to hold the baby. The birth mother may or may not choose to breastfeed the baby immediately after birth. The birth mother may wish to have photos or other mementos of the baby at birth, such as a lock of hair or the baby's footprints. If the birth mom chooses not to hold the baby and the adoptive parents are not present, the baby will be examined in the birthing room by a health-care provider, and then cared for in the hospital nursery.

After the birth, the birth mother will move to a room for her postpartum stay. Often the hospital will make a room available on a different floor than the usual postpartum floor where mothers are together with their babies. The birth mother may be visited in the hospital by a social worker, lawyer, or worker from the adoption agency to start the process for relinquishment of the baby.

With surrogacy, the baby normally goes home from the hospital with the intended parents. With adoption, the baby may go home with the adoptive parents, or the adoptive parents may choose to place the baby in foster care during the waiting period mandated by the location where the baby is born, which may range from two to ninety days. Some adoptive parents decide on foster care so they do not become attached to the baby in the event that the birth mother changes her mind about the adoption.

The doula visits the birth mother postpartum, to talk about her physical and emotional recovery, and her feelings about the baby and the birth, if she wishes. The doula can help the birth mother be aware of symptoms of postpartum depression. Birth mothers can be susceptible to depression during pregnancy, postpartum, and in later years; however, they may also be helped by counselors and support groups specializing in adoption issues. For information about support services for birth mothers and fathers, visit www.birthmother resources.com. (Grandparents and extended family of the birth mother may also experience stress and be in need of counseling and support.)

The doula may also visit the adoptive family postpartum, if it is agreeable to the birth mother. Adoptive or intended parents can be affected by what is becoming known as post-adoptive depression, due to the stressful demands of caring for a newborn along with unresolved feelings about the difficulties of infertility and adoption.

Birth mothers as well as adoptive families may be isolated, or feel a desire for privacy about their situations, and therefore receive less support than people forming their families in more traditional ways. The caring and nonjudgmental support of a doula can be an important resource for these special families. Of course, adoption and surrogacy also bring joy, and a doula can help enhance the positive elements of this experience.

For more information about doulas and surrogacy or adoption, contact the Childbirth and Postpartum Professional Association, at 888-MY-CAPPA or www.cappa.net.

## INTERVIEW YOUR DOULA

Interviewing doulas can be a helpful step in learning to trust your intuition as a mother-to-be:

We found our doula when I was five months pregnant, and then I still needed to decide on a doctor,
because I had mixed feelings about my original obstetrician. Our doula was supportive about my need
to keep looking for a doctor, and I finally found one
when I was almost eight months pregnant. It was the
right decision for me; I had such a positive birth I
decided to become a doula myself. I trusted my intuition about the right doula, and she helped me continue to trust myself until I found the right doctor.

—Akemi, 26, doula, mother of two

You can meet and interview doulas in your home, the
home or office of the doula, at the location of a community
doula program, or another agreed-upon place. Following are
typical interview questions that families ask doulas and which
you may want to ask those you meet:

- Are you available as a doula during the month my baby
  is due?
- Please tell me about your experience as a doula.
- What techniques do you use with women in labor? Do
  you have any specialties (such as massage therapy or
  hypnotherapy)?
- How will you include my partner or loved ones in the
  birth?
- How would you describe your style or manner as a
  doula (quiet, talkative, assertive, cooperative, etc.)?
- What has your experience been at my hospital or with
  my doctor/midwife?
- What are your views about natural childbirth? About
  medications during birth?
- How many meetings will I have with you before and
  after the birth?
- How should I get in touch with you during labor?

- Do you have a backup partner, in case you are not available when I go into labor?
- May I contact your references?
- Do you offer other services, such as postpartum care or lactation counseling?

The doula will also have questions for you, so feel free to think about your answers to some of them ahead of time:

- Have you been learning about birth, or do you need basic information? Have you taken birth classes or read books about birth?
- Who will be with you at your birth? What kind of support would they like to offer, and what kind of support will they need?
- If you have given birth before, what was your experience like?
- How do you wish to handle the potential pain of labor?
- Do you have health concerns or emotional concerns you would like to share? If you have an unusual health condition, can you supply your doula with information about it?

The following advice on choosing your doula is offered by Gina Forbes, CD, the director of ALACE:

> Labor works best when the birthing woman feels safe and supported. In this stress-free environment, oxytocin, the hormone of labor (and love), can function at its peak, making labor efficient and, for many women, joyful or ecstatic. Part of your doula's job is to help you get that oxytocin pumping, and having a trusting, strong connection allows for this process to optimally occur. So don't forget to check in about how you feel about your doula—if she's the right one, you should feel great!

## PAYING FOR YOUR DOULA

Private doulas normally charge a flat fee that covers all (or most) of their services, and includes your birth, regardless of how long it is. The fee also typically includes one or more meetings before and after your birth, and telephone or e-mail discussions.

The initial interview may be free, or the doula may charge a separate fee for it. Occasionally, a doula might charge an extra fee for an extremely long birth, or she might ask you to reimburse her for expenses such as parking at the hospital.

Doula fees can vary widely, based on your geographic location and the experience level of the doula. Typical fees for a newly trained doula in North America are in the range of $300. Fees for an experienced doula start at approximately $600 in smaller towns, and can reach about $2,000 in cities with the highest cost of living, such as San Francisco or New York City.

Doulas in European nations including Belgium, the Czech Republic, Hungary, Portugal, and Spain report fees of approximately €80 to €250 (euros). Fees in countries such as France, Germany, Ireland, the Netherlands, Switzerland, and the United Kingdom are reported at €350 to €1,200.

In recent years, as doulas have become more professionalized, they've strived to set fees that reflect the true value of providing one-on-one care to families, something even most doctors and midwives no longer offer. As respected doula trainer Ilana Stein of New York City remarked, "Being on call is worth its weight in gold." At the same time, doulas have a tradition of aiming to work sensitively with all women regardless of income.

Doulas may offer payment plans or other individualized financial arrangements; if you are in need of this, be sure to inquire with your doula. Doulas-in-training commonly offer their services at a reduced fee or on a volunteer basis, and some experienced doulas also volunteer for clients in need. To find a lower-cost doula, simply ask as you make calls. The ALACE Web site indicates which of its doula members are available to volunteer, at www.alace.org. (Also, some hospitals or community programs offer doula services at no charge, particularly for low-income families.)

If you are placing your baby for adoption in the U.S., the doula's fee may be considered an official health-care expense, to be paid for by the adoptive parents through the adoption agency. In Canada, doula fees currently cannot be paid by the adoptive parents. In these cases, you may inquire with doulas about volunteer services.

## ⟨⟨ BABY GIFT REGISTRIES ⟩⟩

For a creative way to raise money to pay for your doula, use a baby gift registry.

Special Web sites allow you to set up a registry to receive cash gifts from friends and relatives, which you can apply to the cost of your doula. Many family members would be delighted to share the cost of doula services, rather than (or in addition to) another stuffed animal or baby outfit. Not everyone feels comfortable asking for cash, but moms-to-be who do so typically find they can raise at least half the cost of a doula by "registering" for it. Web sites with a cash gifts registry include:

www.felicite.com

www.gogift.com

www.myregistry.com

## INSURANCE COVERAGE FOR DOULAS

Is it possible to use your health insurance to pay for doula services? Maybe. Currently, insurance coverage is usually not automatic, but families can contact their health plans individually and file a claim to attempt to pay for their doula. Those who've done so say the key to requesting and receiving payment from your insurance company is to persist, persist, persist.

Asking your insurance company for payment is not a mysterious process. However, the timing of when you file your claim can be important. It is better to start your claim while you are still pregnant, though you can file it afterward if necessary, according to Marnie Cabezas Skorupa, CPM, owner of an insurance billing company specializing in birth services. In your communications, emphasize the potential for doulas to *save your insurance company money* by reducing expensive medical procedures.

These are the steps to take:

1. Call the customer service number of your insurance company and ask for the name and address where you should submit a claim for maternity care.
2. Ask if your insurance covers birth doulas. If they say no, ask for an "exception" or a "pre-authorization," which they would put in writing.
3. If you are hiring a doula instead of using an epidural, or to help avoid a cesarean, tell your insurance company. Ask how much they pay for these procedures, including the extra days of a hospital stay after a cesarean. Write these numbers down.
4. Before your birth, ask your midwife or doctor for a prescription for a birth doula. This can be in the form of a letter or simply written on a prescription pad.
5. Pay your doula out of pocket and ask her for a receipt or invoice. Her invoice should include the *diagnostic code* for pregnancy and the *treatment code* for doula

services (or the treatment code for "unspecified maternity services"). If your doula is not certain of what these codes should be, ask your insurance company.

6. After your birth, mail your request to your insurance company to reimburse you. Include the doula's invoice and your provider's prescription.

7. With your claim, you can mail copies of research showing the benefits of doulas, such as that found in the Cochrane Collaboration database. Go to the Web site www.cochrane.org, and search for the review titled "Continuous Support for Women during Childbirth."

8. The first time a claim is submitted, it is often automatically rejected, in which case you'll need to file an appeal. Once again, call and ask for the name and address to whom you should send your appeal (this may be a different name than the first time).

9. At this time, you'll need to provide additional supporting documents with your appeal. You can write a letter detailing how you saved your insurance company money by using a doula. If you avoided an epidural or a cesarean, include the costs of these procedures. (In some areas of the U.S. the difference in cost between a vaginal birth and a cesarean has been calculated at over $7,000. Avoiding an epidural can save $1,000 or more.)

10. At your workplace, ask the benefits manager in your human resources office to write a letter to your insurer on your behalf, and include it with your appeal.

11. If your insurer has reimbursed other patients for doulas, you can say so. You can also tell your insurer which other companies have done so. (See below.)

12. You can contact your state insurance commissioner

to assist you, and inform your insurer that you are doing so.

13. Your appeal may be denied, in which case you may appeal a second time. Your first appeal will probably be reviewed by an administrator at the insurance company, while your second appeal may be reviewed by a doctor or nurse. Although this process is tedious, those who work with the insurance industry report that the majority of consumers who make appeals are eventually paid by their insurers.

## INSURERS THAT HAVE PAID FOR DOULAS

We spoke with Debbie Young, the president of DONA International, who was also chair of the DONA Third Party Reimbursement Committee for seven years. Doula advocates are currently working on getting an insurance treatment code established specifically for doula services. (Until now, a code for "unspecified services" has been used.) Once a doula treatment code becomes official, reimbursement for doula services is expected to be easier.

So far, insurance companies have paid for doula services on a case-by-case basis, rather than automatically paying for all doulas. According to information collected by the DONA Third Party Reimbursement Committee, as well as individual doulas we interviewed, insurance companies that have reimbursed for doula care include:

| | |
|---|---|
| Aetna | Humana |
| Baylor Health Care System | Maritime Life |
| Blue Cross and Blue Shield | Oschner HMO |
|     Association | Oxford |
| Cigna | Prudential |
| Elmcare | Travelers |
| Fortis | United Healthcare |
| Great-West Life & Annuity | |

## LOOK WHO'S USING
### ∽ DOULAS NOW ∾

Like everyday moms, celebrities have been discovering the benefits of doulas, too.

Actress and former talk show host Ricki Lake now has a new title: she's been called an "honorary" doula who has learned all she could about birth, and put that to use assisting at the births of friends and creating her 2007 documentary, *The Business of Being Born.* Within one month of its release, nearly one hundred thousand viewers requested the film from www.netflix.com, the online video service. The editor of *Mothering* magazine called it "the best birth film ever made."

The film has also been compared to former vice president Al Gore's *An Inconvenient Truth,* for its scrutiny of maternity care as an industry influenced by monetary and legal concerns, sometimes at the expense of mothers and babies.

But some of the most compelling parts of the film revolve around Lake herself, who appears in the movie naked in the bathtub of her home, giving birth to her second son with support from several providers, including two doulas. In interviews, Lake says the experience was a defining moment in her life, one that taught her the power of her own body, helped her to face hidden ghosts of past abuse, and launched her into a new role as the most well-known spokesperson for empowering birthing women. She has said that the experience healed her in many ways, emotionally and physically, as it began her much-publicized weight loss and new focus on health and fitness.

In the film, Tina Cassidy, author of *Birth: The Surprising History of How We Are Born*, **points out that elective C-sections (those done without a medical reason) gained attention when celebrities such as Victoria "Posh Spice" Beckham signed on for them, a trend that became known as "too posh to push." We hope Lake sparks a countertrend: women calling for more compassionate maternity care that is focused on what's best for them and their babies, rather than legal and business interests.**

Some famous folks reported to have hired doulas include:

- Samantha Bee and Jason Jones, actors
- Rachael Beck and Ian Stenlake, actors
- Cindy Crawford, model
- Diane Farr, actor
- Joely Fisher, actor
- Maggie Gyllenhaal and Peter Sarsgaard, actors
- Maria Hinojosa, news show host
- Tina Holmes, actor
- Rob Lowe, actor
- Eric Mabius, actor
- Elle Macpherson, model/actor
- Tonya Pinkins, actor
- Kelly Ripa, talk show host
- Kate Winslet, actor
- Jaret Wright, former N.Y. Yankees starting pitcher

6

# DOULAS AND MEDICAL PROVIDERS

Many doctors, midwives, and nurses see doulas as another set of helping hands and welcome them into the delivery room. But like any professionals who work together in close proximity under intense and often stressful conditions, obstetric providers and doulas can sometimes find themselves at odds. In the past few years, as more women have begun to rely on doulas for emotional support during childbirth, strong teams have developed in some hospitals, with all of the practitioners working collaboratively and in sync.

Doctors and midwives who are caring for more than one laboring mother at the same time, for example, can rely on doulas, who provide continuous support, for important updates, says Beth Hardiman, an obstetrician/gynecologist at Mount Auburn Hospital in Cambridge, Massachusetts. She says the doula can help catch her up on what's going on in the delivery room. "She can tell me what's working, what's not, whether the laboring mom has been in the tub or walking around," Dr. Hardiman says. "The doula can be a support person for the whole team, so that no one—the partner, the doctor, or the nurses—feels overwhelmed or overburdened."

But doulas' increased visibility in hospitals has sometimes led to tension over turf. This is a normal phenomenon that tends to happen whenever a new profession begins to establish itself. Of course, you would prefer to avoid tension in the delivery room. So how can you ensure that your birth team really is a team?

## STRAIGHT TALK

Some tension can be avoided if each of your providers has been clearly informed about your wishes for birth. In most situations, doctors and midwives, nurses and doulas perform specific jobs that are fairly well defined. There is some overlap, however, and that's when conflict might arise if, for instance, you've told your doctor or midwife something about your desires for birth and haven't informed your doula, or vice versa.

Mothers sometimes wonder about whether a laboring woman even needs a doula if she is giving birth with a midwife. Since hospital-based midwives have many of the same constraints as doctors, such as shift changes and group practices that leave the laboring mother unsure of who will actually deliver her baby, we think the answer is an emphatic yes. (Doulas can also help at home births, particularly in the early stages of labor, before the midwife or doctor arrives.)

Doulas do not replace nurses or other medical staff.

Doulas will not make decisions on your behalf or intervene in your clinical care. They simply provide information—most of it in discussions *before* labor about options and choices and expectations—and emotional support. As one doula put it, "I am there to slow down time so *you* have time to make your own decisions." She added, "I want mothers to be active decision-makers in their births."

The best way to lay the groundwork for a positive group effort in the delivery room is to talk frankly to your doula and your doctor or midwife well before birth. Ask your provider specifically how she feels about doulas. How many births has she been to with a doula present? Does she have any questions or concerns about doulas?

Some hospitals supply a doula referral list to pregnant women. These lists are generally not all-inclusive and are simply a starting-off point that includes some of the local doulas who doctors or midwives know or have worked with. If your doula is not on this list, don't fret. But do mention her name to your provider, and you might choose to bring her in for one of your prenatal visits.

If you want a doula present because you wish for a VBAC, or you want to deliver twins without an epidural, or if you had an unpleasant experience during a previous birth and want something different, be specific with your provider. You might need to consider looking for another doctor if your current provider is not at least open to discussing different approaches.

While interviewing potential doulas, you should also be specific. Ask how she might handle a situation in which she and the doctor or midwife have differing opinions. Ask about her experience supporting women who opted for pain medications or who had C-sections. If the answer isn't satisfactory or you detect a rigidity that doesn't fit with your own beliefs, don't hire her. Remember, your doula is all your own so think about what type of person might make the best match. You may want the most assertive doula in town, or want a doula with a strong personality that matches your own. Or you might want a doula who will be very cooperative with your caregivers and not challenge them.

Once you choose a doula who you really feel comfortable with, continue to talk about this topic. Has she ever attended a birth with your doctor? What was that like? Has she been welcomed at your hospital? Or ignored? Remember, most of the discussions you will have with your doula about your general wishes and preferences for birth will take place well before labor begins. The more strategizing you can do beforehand, the smoother things will likely be in the heat of the moment.

A doula explains, "Have I helped change the direction of things in labor? Yes. But not because I've been adversarial. I've done it by asking questions, and by reminding the mother of what she indicated her wishes were prenatally."

> I'm a doctor, but I used a doula to help with the births of both my children because I know doulas have a unique role during labor. I hadn't spent that much time with my OB—she was part of a group practice—but my doula was someone I'd built an intimate trust with. And she'd also developed a great relationship with my husband, who bombarded her with e-mails and questions before birth. He relied on her to help him through my labor over twenty-four hours.
>
> During that time, my OB was in and out, tracking my progress, but the doula was with us every minute—for all the blood, sweat, and tears. When the baby needed medical attention right after her birth, the doula stepped aside and let the doctors do their thing to make sure the baby was breathing properly. Everything turned out fine, but it really became clear what the different roles were. They

> complemented each other's work and together en-
> hanced the experience for me.
>
> —Lydia, 40, radiologist, mother of two

From the doctors' perspective, sometimes problems can surface when doulas step far beyond their roles as support people. Doulas, however, say they must work hard to balance the hospital staff's institutional authority with women's wishes.

Again, Dr. Hardiman says the best doulas work to remind women and their partners of what they had wanted. But if things change during the course of labor—and often they do—doulas help reframe or reset expectations, so ultimately there can be some acceptance of the path that birth takes.

Dr. William Camann, director of obstetric anesthesia services at Brigham and Women's Hospital in Boston, has been trying for several years to bridge the gap between doctors, nurses, and doulas. For instance, he says, he has invited doulas to remain with the laboring mother in the operating room during a C-section, and to stay by the mother's side during the insertion of the needle for an epidural. He says when he can, he tries to walk the doula through the entire procedure. "How can a doula explain and support a woman through an epidural if they don't know the procedure or don't know what the needle looks like?" Dr. Camann says. "I think it's totally compatible for a woman to get pain medication and have a doula."

## THE DOULA PERSPECTIVE

Jane Look, a veteran doula in Massachusetts, says when she first started out in the late 1980s, doctors simply ignored her. But over time she won the respect of even the most conservative doctors and nurses. She says when mothers decide to give birth in a hospital, they've already accepted the institution's rules on some level, and it's important for the doula to understand this.

Joyce Kimball, another doula, says, "My job as a doula is to care for the mom and dad." So she tries to frame all of her communication with that intention—of caring for the family's physical and emotional well-being. "I have said things like, 'It seems to really sting when fingers are on her perineum while she's pushing. Can we just put a cloth there?' Or, 'It seems like her back is sore because she's arching while pushing. Can she lie on her side?' As long as I read Mom well, offer suggestions and changes for a reason, and don't just demand or fight, the OBs are happy to have me there."

A Rhode Island doula, Judy Batson, says when attending births at a hospital, she is always mindful that she is on the nurses' turf. "I am respectful to the nurses and show that I will do whatever I can to help relieve them of mundane duties such as fetching fluids and snacks. I do not speak for my client directly to the nurse or the other medical professionals. Helping the client learn how to ask questions is one of the things I do when we meet prenatally. I encourage my clients to ask the nurses questions. Most nurses are really into providing patient information and education."

## WORKING FOR YOU

When a true spirit of teamwork is established, the laboring mother benefits. You can freely turn to your loved ones or any one of your caregivers, whether it's the doctor, midwife, nurse, or doula at different moments of labor to get what you need. Carolyn Ogren, a doula trainer and former labor and delivery nurse, recalled such a birth where the mother "leaned on each one of us when she needed a certain skill, talent, or expertise that she thought we had to offer. She might check in with each of us to see who had the most valuable thing for her to choose. Or she may have been looking for the reassurance that we all had the same answer to a question."

7

# WHEN SHOULD YOU REALLY GO TO THE HOSPITAL IN LABOR?

*My contractions began on a Thursday, and my daughter was not born until the following Thursday. I spoke to my doula most days that week. She explained right away that I might have a gradual labor, and that some women are surprised at how hard it can feel to be in limbo like that. She was right—I burst into tears a few times that week, and went to the hospital three times, only to have to go home. But when labor finally kicked in strongly in the middle of Wednesday night, my doula encouraged me not to doubt my judgment about what I was feeling. We headed to the hospital, and I gave birth to my daughter four hours later.*

—Leslie, 37, engineer, mother of one

The beginning of labor is a mystery; we normally do not know when it will happen, and science has not figured out why labor starts when it does. It is also a moment of great personal meaning to the woman entering motherhood, as well as a time of vulnerability. Since labor may last from several hours to several days, how will you know exactly when to leave for your hospital or birth center (if you are not having a home birth)?

First-time mothers are not expected to be experts at diagnosing whether they are in active labor, and many women do arrive at the hospital earlier than necessary. For some mothers, being at the place where they will give birth is a relief and they eagerly agree to be admitted, even if they could have stayed home several hours longer. Others feel embarrassed, frustrated, or disappointed that they misjudged labor, especially if they are advised to go home.

Is the timing of when to arrive at the hospital so important? Many first-time mothers worry about *not* getting to the hospital in time to give birth, but this is rarely the problem they'll face in reality. If a woman feels she cannot manage early labor without an epidural, she will of course have to go to the hospital in order to receive one. If the mother experiences abnormal symptoms such as heavy bleeding, she will need to seek care in the hospital.

For a healthy pregnant woman having her first labor, there are usually advantages to delaying admission to the hospital. Many doctors candidly admit that women interested in natural childbirth are better served by staying home longer, because once they are admitted, medical procedures are likely to be used simply because the equipment is there and providers are familiar with it.

How can we best preserve a woman's chance to labor without unnecessary interventions? In the larger picture, the solution should not be to guard and keep her away from the hospital. She has entrusted her care to the hospital, and she should feel safe and comfortable going there, regardless of the timing of it. But in today's maternity-care climate, pregnant women (and doulas) often find themselves in the position of trying to shield the mother from entering the hospital too soon.

According to the Cochrane Collaboration, women who

arrive at the hospital "too" early are indeed subject to more medical interventions, including more cesareans. (The top reason for cesareans today is not a medical emergency, it is simply a slower than average labor; see chapter 8 for more information.)

## EXPECTATIONS AND REALITY

Little research exists about women's experiences of early labor before they get to the hospital. However, a 2006 pilot study in the *Journal of Midwifery & Women's Health* drew the following conclusions: Mothers often plan for and idealize childbirth, but when faced with the reality of early labor, they may feel confused about what is happening and when to go to the hospital. This uncertainty in early labor may undermine their confidence, satisfaction, and even the smooth progress of their labors. The authors conclude it would be beneficial to have a system in place to provide reassurance, support, and feedback in early labor at home. Although the study did not focus on this solution, the use of a doula is currently one of the only available options for receiving such support during these important early hours.

The difference between your familiar home environment and the hospital setting can be an important factor in your emotional and physical comfort level. At home you'll have the freedom to move from room to room, go outside for a walk, or take a car ride to distract yourself (with someone else in the driver's seat). In the hospital, you will be mainly confined to your delivery room, many of which are so small they seem not to have been designed with labor in mind.

The familiarity of home can give you a sense of confidence and mastery over your environment. Have you ever been to an important meeting in an unfamiliar location (for example a job interview, blind date, business meeting, or even interviewing your doula at her office)? Upon arriving, you may not have been able to concentrate on the meeting itself, because you were busy adjusting to the new surroundings, and it may have taken time to regain your confidence about participating in the meeting.

A hospital room is unfamiliar, containing medical equipment that may look complicated or intimidating, and staffed by strangers who move quickly and assuredly through their environment. Social scientists who study modern birthing customs have documented the elaborate "rituals" that take place in delivery wards. Many of these customs are necessary, of course, to greet the woman, settle her into her room, and evaluate whether she and her baby are in good health. But these rituals may also serve to suggest that a mother lacks control in labor, an event where she already feels highly vulnerable. Doctors, midwives, and nurses convey a sense of authority simply by being more comfortable in a hospital setting than the parents-to-be.

Other conditions within a hospital that might affect your comfort and coping abilities include a lack of locks on the doors, staff coming and going without knocking, doors rarely being closed behind staff, a lack of labor comfort tools such as bathtubs or stereos to play music for relaxation, rules that limit visitors of your own choosing, rules against using cell phones to stay in touch with others, the restriction of food or food being unavailable even if it is permitted, beds and showers that are not large enough for a partner to join you, and being attached to equipment that restricts freedom of movement.

Privacy, low lighting, and quiet allow for the smooth unfolding of labor for humans, like any other mammals. The

World Health Organization recommends that sounds in patients' rooms be kept below thirty to forty decibels, but studies show that average noise levels in most hospitals are double that.

Fathers and loved ones are not always adequately acknowledged and included within the hospital. On the other hand, loved ones are often expected to look after the laboring woman without guidance when medical staff leave the room. Research from Dr. Kennell and the Klauses shows that fathers increasingly move away from the laboring woman as labor gets more intense, when complicated scenarios occur in labor, when hospital staff interact with the mother in an authoritative way, or even when staff simply enter the room.

Staying home longer will extend the hours you have access to the comforts and freedoms of home. When you do arrive at the hospital, one way to ease the transition is to bring items that provide you with a sense of familiarity and comfort. Unpack these items right away so they are not forgotten and they are available to use throughout labor. These items may include such things as a portable stereo, food, a framed photograph from home, earplugs, and a sleep mask.

## ☙ THE PURPOSE OF TRIAGE ❧

One way to manage the uncertainty of early labor is to think of your first visit to the hospital as a time to be *evaluated,* not necessarily admitted. You will want to be ready with your suitcase in case you are admitted, but don't plan on definitely staying unless active labor is confirmed. It is completely all right for you to be incorrect about whether you are in active labor! This is exactly the reason that hospital triage rooms exist.

You will normally not have to wait long to see a caregiver in triage. Your midwife or doctor will check vital signs such as your blood pressure and the baby's heartbeat, which can help reassure you that if you have to go home, it is considered safe to do so. In the U.S., most providers will want to perform a pelvic exam to see if your cervix is opening, a sign of active labor. (These exams may be helpful when deciding whether you should stay at the hospital, but they can be risky if your water has broken; this will be discussed further in the next chapter.)

## IS IT REALLY TIME?

Most providers ask mothers to use the following formula: "When contractions are *three to five* minutes apart for *one* hour, lasting *one* minute each, come to the hospital." (This is sometimes known as the 3-1-1 rule, or the 5-1-1 rule.) These are helpful guidelines to start with; however, we'd like to offer more complete suggestions. Some women have normal labors in which they feel contractions every five minutes for an entire day, but their contractions are mild enough that the cervix is not opening yet, and they're not approaching the middle or end of labor. What can parents and labor assistants do in these situations?

One of the first tasks of labor is simply learning how to tell when the mother is having a contraction. In most cases, it will be clear to the woman herself when each cramping sensation begins and ends. (Occasionally the symptoms of very early labor are so vague that it takes a few hours to realize what is happening, but eventually it will become obvious to the woman.) It also becomes the task of her partner or support person to recognize when she is having a contraction.

At the beginning of labor, a woman can simply tell her support person, "I'm having a contraction now." This is a time for the support person to stop talking, watch and notice how the mother is behaving, and look for opportunities to offer comfort. Quiet words of encouragement such as "good job," along with gentle touch on areas such as the mother's back, are helpful as you learn to recognize when she is having a contraction. Ask her occasionally if she would like you to change the words or the touch you're using, so you know what is helpful to her.

Loved ones, notice how the mother's behavior changes during contractions: she may close her eyes, take a deep breath or sigh loudly, or shift repeatedly to the position that feels most comfortable to her. As the hours pass, watch for her signs. When you have started to figure out what she looks like during contractions, you can begin to ask her, "Are you having one now?" Once you have been correct about this a few times, it is not necessary to ask her every time (this could become irritating). Simply quiet down and offer support during each one. Women and their loved ones learn how to be in labor by doing it, developing routines that work for them and repeating them throughout the entire birth.

Remember, labor is about the pregnant woman! Both partners may be filled with excitement, nervousness, the need to get bags ready to go, and as the hours continue, boredom or a desire for distractions such as watching television or talking. Early labor may last a long time. You'll need to strike a balance between finding activities to pass the time and focusing on what the mother is going through. When a father or support person learns to notice the mother's contractions, the two of them can work more harmoniously together for the whole labor. Even if you don't yet have experience with birth, this can be learned in your first labor.

———

Parents often get the message that they should time every contraction with a watch. Sometimes doulas arrive at a birth and discover their clients have written down the time of every contraction on many pages of paper!

Timing contractions can help give you a sense of some control during an unfamiliar process. However, it's not mandatory to clock them, and we encourage you to leave your watch aside most of the time. For example, you might choose to notice the time of contractions for half an hour, simply to get a sense of whether they're twelve minutes apart or five minutes apart. You can do this occasionally throughout the day. But you'll also want to get a sense of contractions simply by feeling and watching them.

First labors usually start out mild and slow, gradually becoming intense and more rapid. After several hours pass, you'll be able to use your own intuition to say, "These are definitely stronger than what I felt this morning." Loved ones will be able to draw the same conclusions by watching the woman's behavior. You'll be able to *see* when contractions are significantly longer, stronger, and closer together. The difference will be dramatic. With a first labor, you may need to let most of the entire day go by before you notice any real changes.

Watching what contractions look and feel like offers benefits over timing and writing them all down. The mother learns to trust her own intuition about what she is feeling in labor, a highly instinctive process. Partners also learn to become more intuitive about birth. These kinds of observational skills will be valuable in the early days and months of parenting, when once again your instincts will be of paramount importance.

---

Returning to the 3-1-1 formula, probably the most important element of the equation is that it's usually necessary for contractions to be a full one minute long. (This is *along with* contractions coming three to five minutes apart.) If it seems that contractions are indeed one minute long, but they're only coming every ten minutes, it's not likely that labor is active. Also, contractions that are five minutes apart but only last a few seconds are not likely to be active labor. It may take hours of patience before every contraction lasts this long.

## ᕙ CAN YOU TALK? ᕗ

Many providers and childbirth classes advise women to wait to leave home until they feel unable to talk *during* contractions. But often, this is still too early to go. At some point, the mother will begin to feel she's lost interest in talking *between* contractions as well. Experienced doulas have found this to be a better indicator that labor is entering the active phase. At this point, contractions will be close enough together, and long enough, that keeping up with conversation is not really comfortable anymore. Once you've been feeling this way for an hour or two, go ahead to your birth place. For a first baby, these signs usually indicate the beginning of active labor, not the end, and you should still have plenty of time to settle in to the hospital or birth center without missing your chance to get there in time.

Occasionally, a sign of middle or advanced labor may be an early urge to push, including feelings of rectal pressure or involuntary grunting sounds in the mother. Most first-time mothers will not feel this at all while they're home awaiting active labor. But sometimes, a baby who is situated in a low position will stimulate these sensations in the mother. This usually does not mean the baby is about to be pushed out, but it is a signal to head for the hospital in case labor is getting closer to the end. If you are having your second or subsequent vaginal birth, pushing will not take as long, so head out right away if these sensations begin.

If your water breaks before contractions begin, you will be asked to call your caregiver. Different providers have different protocols about when to be admitted to the hospital under this circumstance, and debate exists about this topic. (See chapter 8 for more information.)

Finally, an important sign that it's time to go to the hospital is your intuition. If you sense that you need to be in the place where you will give birth, even if contractions do not appear to indicate active labor, follow these instincts. Your body and intuition may signal that this will be an unusually short labor, or that something else is happening which makes it appropriate to be at the hospital sooner. Or you might have a strong psychological need to settle in at the hospital and put thoughts of getting there behind you.

--------

The suggestions we've made so far mainly apply to first-time mothers, who can expect to have longer labors. Mothers having a second or subsequent baby sometimes have the opposite issues; they need help getting to the hospital in a timely manner. Arrangements to care for older children need to be enacted. Active labor often begins within the first couple of hours for experienced moms, and it is usually appropriate to head to the hospital near the beginning of labor, when contractions are about five to seven minutes apart.

Some mothers realize they could have stayed home much longer during their first birth, and therefore decide they want to do so during their second. They may feel strongly about this, but in fact persuasion may be needed to help them recognize that second labors necessitate going to the hospital sooner, not later.

## ABNORMAL SYMPTOMS IN EARLY LABOR

Research supports the safety of staying home in early labor for healthy pregnant women. However, the following symptoms may indicate that labor is proceeding abnormally. Contact or go to your hospital if you experience the following:

- You have bleeding as heavy as a menstrual period.
- You have pain in the abdomen *between* contractions.
- The baby is not making its normal movements.
- When your water breaks, it is green or brown rather than clear.
- When your water breaks, you feel the baby's umbilical cord slip down in your vagina.
- You have an intuition that something is wrong.

## SUPPORT FOR EARLY LABOR

How can a doula help while you are still at home? Most doctors and midwives request that you call by the time contractions are about five minutes apart. Your doula, on the other hand, will usually ask you to call her at the start of very early labor, so she can finish her activities and be ready to leave on a moment's notice later on.

After the first phone call, the doula will be available to talk regularly in early labor, which at times may be needed every hour or two. A mother may feel hesitant to call her provider or the hospital that often, but a doula can help parents feel they are not alone. This can be very calming, especially if early labor lasts for several days.

Sizing up the progress of labor is an advanced skill. Some experienced doulas can help give feedback about when labor is active enough to go to the hospital by taking stock of the mother's behavior; these doulas can provide a valuable service by doing so.

Many doulas are not experienced enough to judge the subtleties of active labor. However, newer doulas may be more available to come to a client's home and provide hands-on support in early labor. Their goal is to help decrease nervousness for the parents for a few hours, and they can also gain experience judging the appearance of labor.

Other doulas join their clients at home with the *intention* of supporting them in remaining there longer. These doulas may find themselves spending many hours offering comfort at home, and even sleeping at the client's house in order to help extend the mother's time there.

However, experienced doulas may choose not to offer support in the home, feeling it is best for parents—as well as doulas—to rest in early labor, and to save their stamina for the hospital when it is needed most.

A small number of doulas have completed additional training, usually as nurses or student midwives, and are skilled in performing exams to confirm the cervix is opening before leaving for the hospital. One of the doula organizations, DONA International, feels a doula's role is not to perform these kinds of measurements. On the other hand, certain doulas who are qualified in these skills do choose to incorporate them in their services as doulas, for mothers who request them. (Doulas do not perform cervical exams in the hospital.)

When labor begins, how do you know whether your partner or support person should stay home from work, if labor could take days? If your partner has the option, we recommend that he or she stays home. This way, the two of you will not be preoccupied with anxiety about what is happening with the other person. It's even possible that a mother might unconsciously slow down her labor while waiting for her partner to return. By staying home together, you may help prevent these kinds of delays in labor.

If it would not be possible for your main support person to remain home from work for days of early labor, be prepared with a list of other friends or relatives you can call. Don't be shy about asking them to come over and keep you company. Labor is a time of vulnerability, and there's no better occasion in life to ask for the support you need.

You may want to be ready with relaxing activities you can do to pass the time in early labor, when you'll still be alert to the world around you, and before you need to use coping techniques. Set aside some videos to watch, or get the listings for your local movie theater, which some laboring women have been known to do. It's fine to do things outside, as long as you take it easy and don't exhaust yourself before active labor. Take a walk in your neighborhood or at a favorite nearby place such as a beach or lake. (One couple we knew wanted to go out in a canoe, but that type of activity is really too ambitious for labor!)

Eat normally while you are still at home so you'll have the fuel to keep going when labor gets more intense hours later. Play cards or board games. Feel free to call and chat with friends and relatives (but just be aware they'll probably call you repeatedly for updates once they know you're in labor). Read books and magazines, take naps and showers, and do whatever light activities feel helpful. And if you're partnered, take some luxurious time to cuddle one last time while it's life with just the two of you.

Like Leslie, the mother whose story opened this chapter, remember that a slow early labor can be exciting as well as nerve-racking. Being sent home from the hospital can leave parents feeling insecure about how they'll cope for more hours alone. Check in with your doula for support. Even if she does not usually come to the home in labor, she might be willing to stop by and give you her encouragement in person.

Be sure to stay well rested; if it is the middle of the night, you can use techniques such as taking a long bath or drinking a glass of wine to temporarily stop early labor. (See "How to Sleep in Early Labor" in chapter 9.) Or use lovemaking to boost your spirits if you get sent home. If you feel emotional about the uncertainty of early labor, let yourself cry or otherwise express your feelings. It's OK to weep with frustration about labor, or with nervousness about becoming a mother. Remind yourself that these feelings are completely normal, and even to be expected during a long early labor.

The start of labor is the beginning of your rite of passage into motherhood. Use this time to listen to your body and your baby, learn about your contractions and your unique labor patterns, and begin to find the comfort techniques that work best for you; the way early labor is handled can have an effect on your entire birth.

## IN REVIEW:
## WHEN TO GO TO THE
## ☙ HOSPITAL IN LABOR ❧

- When contractions are *three to five* minutes apart, lasting *one* minute each, for *one* hour (the 3-1-1 rule)
- For mothers having their second or subsequent baby, when contractions are five to seven minutes apart
- When you can no longer talk *between* contractions, not just *during* contractions
- If you feel the urge to push
- If you have heavy bleeding, pain between contractions, if green or brown fluid is leaking from your vagina, if the baby is not moving, or the baby's umbilical cord slips out of your vagina
- If your intuition tells you to go, regardless of other signs
- When in doubt, or if you are high risk, consult with your medical provider

*From* **The Doula Guide to Birth** *by Lowe and Zimmerman. May be copied for individual use.*

# 8

# LABOR IS NOT ABOUT DILATION

*When I arrived at the hospital in labor with my doula, the doctor said my cervix was dilated about 6 centimeters. And it stayed that way for another twenty-four hours. In that time, many doctors, nurses, and medical students came in and out of my room to check on me. The youngest doctor seemed anxious, but everyone else said my baby's heartbeat was doing fine, and if what I was doing was working for me, to keep going until he was born, which I did.*

—Dvora, 24, receptionist, mother of one

In today's maternity care, labor is often described in terms of *dilation*. This means that as the hours of labor pass, a doctor, midwife, or nurse measures the opening of a woman's uterus (her cervix). Dilation is said to go from 0 to 10 centimeters wide, although these are not exact measurements. In reality a fully open cervix is somewhere between 9 and 12 centimeters; the size of the baby's head determines how wide the mother stretches open.

How is dilation detected? In countries including the U.S. and the U.K., caregivers perform many pelvic exams on a woman in labor to try to guess dilation. These estimates vary from provider to provider, and can even change for the same doctor upon doing a repeat exam. (Exams in labor are normally performed just with the provider's fingers, not a speculum.) Several inventors have also tried to patent machines that attach to the cervix to measure dilation, but so far, these devices haven't ever become popular.

There is currently a large amount of handling of a woman's vagina in labor by her caregivers. The frequency of exams is not the same everywhere, but on average, providers may perform exams in labor every two hours, and with almost *every* contraction during pushing. This can result in dozens of pelvic exams in a single labor!

The practice of frequent exams overlooks one of the more important principles of facilitating a smooth labor: humans, like other animals, do better during birth when they are not disturbed by outsiders. It is hard to think of an activity that would disturb a woman's comfort and concentration in labor more than a pelvic exam (usually made more uncomfortable by placing the woman on her back, and sometimes by performing exams during, rather than between, contractions).

Providers do not always ask mothers for express consent to do every vaginal exam. However, you do have the right to negotiate about how often you will be examined, or even to possibly eliminate vaginal exams in labor.

In theory, other information may be gathered with these exams, such as whether the baby's head has rotated into the best position for birth. This too is highly subject to error; doctors are incorrect about determining the baby's head position almost 70 percent of the time, according to a 2003 study in the *Journal of Maternal-Fetal & Neonatal Medicine*. Providers also use exams to judge whether the baby has descended in the mother's vagina. In labor, however, the skin on a baby's head undergoes some normal swelling, known as *caput*. Because of caput, measuring descent with pelvic exams is less accurate, too.

There are several important things that checking dilation does not reveal. It does not tell us whether the baby is healthy. It never tells us how much longer labor will be. And it does not necessarily tell us whether a woman's body is making normal progress in labor, although trying to judge *progress* is the main reason providers are trained to perform these exams. But as we'll explore further in this chapter, the number of hours it takes for dilation to change can vary greatly from woman to woman.

A mother may be as curious as her provider for some sign about how much closer she is getting to the end of labor. But just as often, a woman says she feels discouraged to learn her cervix is only slightly more open, or has not changed, or is possibly even smaller than the last time it was checked. Yet all of those scenarios can happen in the course of normal labor.

Some women may find pelvic exams in labor to be intrusive, while others are less bothered by them. Your response to pelvic exams in a doctor's office, or to the idea of an unfamiliar provider touching your genitals, can tell you how you may respond in labor. Of course, if an epidural is in place, you'll feel less physical discomfort during exams. Women who have experienced sexual abuse may have stronger feelings about receiving exams. If you have a personal preference for as little intrusion as possible, this too is a legitimate reason to request that exams not be performed, if there are no other medical problems.

Many women are unaware that vaginal exams can be declined, and therefore providers may rarely hear women do so. Even when they are declined, a provider's impulse to do exams can be strong. Asking for "no exams" or being specific about the number you prefer will probably be more helpful than requesting "minimal" exams, because one doctor's minimum may be two exams, another's may be twenty.

If you want this option, you may have to remind your providers multiple times, but the effort can be worthwhile. In addition to preserving personal comfort, eliminating vaginal exams can help prevent serious problems by greatly reducing the chances of contracting a harmful infection, or even having an unnecessary induction or cesarean due to infections caused by exams, as we'll discuss further.

———————

In labor, the first vaginal exam is typically performed when a mother arrives at the hospital, or when her midwife or doctor arrives for a home birth. Many women will find out at this point that their cervix is at the beginning of dilation, likely estimated to be open 2 or 3 centimeters. On the one hand, this is great news; most hours in labor are usually spent getting to that point! On the other hand, a mother often hears this as discouraging, considering she may have been waiting at home for a while, and labor still has to last until her cervix is 10 centimeters.

If you partake in this initial exam, we encourage you to *expect* a small amount of dilation; if this exam shows more dilation, think of it as "gravy," or a bonus. Also, remember that active labor will go faster later. However, if labor is still mild enough or your cervix has not begun to open yet, you may have hours or an entire day ahead of you before you are considered to be in "real" labor. Your provider may offer you the option of going home, and it can be to your advantage to do so: studies show that women who are admitted to the hospital early are subject to more interventions, including more cesareans.

If this is your second vaginal birth, you are likely to be in active labor nearly from the beginning, and this initial exam may be less useful to you altogether.

## IS SLOW DILATION BAD FOR YOU?

Midwives and doctors have probably known about using vaginal exams in labor for centuries. The idea of judging "labor progress" came about after the development of the Friedman curve, a chart that relates the length of labor to the amount of dilation. Dr. Emanuel Friedman created this chart in the 1950s, simply as a way to study average lengths of labor in women. Today this curve is being used by doctors to decide whether a labor has gone on too long. In fact, the most common diagnosis leading to a cesarean now is not a medical emergency; it's a vague condition called *failure to progress.*

### ⤳ EMERGENCY CESAREANS? ⤳

Many people use the term *emergency cesarean* to describe the operation anytime it is used, and indeed, this major surgery was once reserved only for truly dire situations. But today, the Cochrane Collaboration reports that cesareans are performed for genuine medical emergencies, such as abnormal bleeding or immediate danger to the baby, in less than 3 percent of births. Now cesareans are mainly being used to treat slower labors.

In the event of a true emergency, hospital staff will refer to a *stat cesarean* or a *crash cesarean.*

Cesarean rates are at an all-time high of over 31 percent in the United States, and over 23 percent in nations including Australia, Canada, and the U.K. The U.S. has one of the highest

## ☁ EMERGENCY CESAREANS? ☁

*(continued from previous page)*

cesarean rates in the world—with these surgeries mostly being performed on healthy mothers and healthy babies—yet ranks nearly last in preventing infant mortality among developed nations. Hence the controversy about how commonly they are being used.

In contrast, the most fascinating example of a very low cesarean rate is found at The Farm in Summertown, Tennessee. The Farm was founded by Stephen and Ina May Gaskin as a large commune in the 1970s. Mrs. Gaskin and other women at The Farm taught themselves to become midwives and have delivered over two thousand babies, 96 percent without medical help, as documented by researchers in the *American Journal of Public Health.*

By relying heavily on human support and reserving obstetric intervention only for emergencies, The Farm has managed to produce a cesarean rate of an astonishing 1.4 percent, along with an infant mortality rate lower than the U.S. national average. And "failure to progress" is a virtually nonexistent diagnosis at The Farm.

Newer studies dispute the Friedman curve as a yardstick by which to diagnose whether there is a problem in a woman's length of labor—and Dr. Friedman himself states he never intended his work to be used for that purpose. In 2003, *Journal Watch Women's Health* published a commentary on the current research, titled "The Friedman Curve: An Obsolete Approach to Labor Assessment."

In the 1950s, Friedman said the average active labor (from

about 4 to 10 centimeters dilation) was a mere two and a half hours. In the 1970s, he revised his curve to say active labor was almost twice that long. Every decade since the original Friedman curve, major changes have occurred in the types of medication used on laboring women. Earlier pain drugs are no longer available, epidural use has climbed, and Pitocin rates have gone up and down; all of these factors have affected the length of "normal" labors.

Multiple studies in the 1990s and 2000s produced different data than Friedman's. Research in the *Journal of Perinatology,* involving 3,984 women who received no drugs in labor, found an "average" active labor three hours longer than Friedman's, as well as safe outcomes with active labors as long as nineteen hours.

*Williams Obstetrics,* the most widely used textbook for obstetricians in the world, makes the following statement within its pages in bold emphasis:

**When time breaches in normal labor boundaries are the only pregnancy complications, interventions other than cesarean delivery must be considered before resorting to this method of delivery for failure to progress.**

Although physicians have been urged not to consider slow dilation alone to be a medical problem, in a 2005 practice bulletin the American College of Obstetricians and Gynecologists estimated that 60 percent of cesareans are based on a diagnosis of failure to progress.

Many doulas propose another approach to managing longer labors, rather than placing such heavy emphasis on dilation: *simply put, be patient.* And science is backing up the same idea: that in general, labor is safer for babies and mothers when it is not placed on a timeline or forced to hurry along.

In hospitals, the most common treatment for a slower labor is to speed it up with Pitocin. Partly to counteract the reliance on drugs, many people have searched for alternative ways to hasten labor, including herbs, acupuncture, and changing the mother's position in complicated ways. We'd like to point out, though, that the best approach may be to respect the natural rhythms of labor, do nothing to interfere, and help the mother *rest*.

Natural oxytocin is not produced in a constant, steady stream. Pitocin, however, is used at a steadily rising rate in labor, creating a more aggressive contraction pattern. Doctors may have begun to expect natural labors to perform like Pitocin-influenced labors, which is not realistic and not necessarily healthiest for babies and mothers.

In natural labors, contractions and dilation normally speed up, slow down, plateau, stop, and speed up again. And while it may seem that the use of Pitocin would result in shorter births than natural labors, studies have shown that the presence of a doula, or preserving the mother's freedom to sit up and walk around, may result in shorter labors than those with Pitocin.

───────

What are reasons that labor might go more slowly? In many cases, longer labors are simply healthy variations on normal birth.

Researchers estimate 30 to 50 percent of slow labors may be due to a cervix that is more firm or rigid, not due to "inadequate contractions" that need Pitocin. For some women, in the last weeks of pregnancy, the cervix becomes soft and thin in preparation for birth; for other women, the cervix does not thin (*efface*) until labor starts, and studies show their births are longer because they must accomplish this in early labor.

Women with a history of using birth control pills may have a firmer cervix that dilates more slowly. Other women may have scarring on the cervix that takes longer to dilate. Scarring may be a result of procedures and events including:

1. Removal of tissue after a miscarriage (D&C)
2. Previous births in which the cervix sustained tiny tears during pushing
3. Abortion
4. Insertion of an IUD
5. Treatments for abnormal pap smears or genital warts, such as cryosurgery (freezing)
6. Taking a biopsy from the cervix or inside the uterus
7. Removal of polyps

These scars are not otherwise harmful in labor, but they may require more hours or even days of contractions to soften and dilate this tougher tissue. Not all women with scars will necessarily have longer labors, though.

In 2008, a study in the *New England Journal of Medicine* analyzed the births of 27,472 mothers in London. The length of each woman's cervix was measured by ultrasound during her pregnancy. The researchers found the cesarean rate was highest among women who simply had a longer cervix and therefore took longer to dilate. They concluded: "The increased risk of cesarean delivery was attributable to procedures performed for poor progress in labor."

For some mothers, slower dilation may be what is normal for their bodies:

> I prepared excitedly for a vaginal birth after cesarean. But my second labor was like my first, with dilation slowing down late in labor, and my doctor began suggesting another cesarean. I felt I was really losing control and losing hope. Then my doula said she'd seen other women in my situation give birth vaginally by waiting longer. The doctor was open to trying this approach.
>
> I got an epidural to help me relax and calm down, which was different from my first birth, where an

epidural was used just to prepare for a cesarean. A couple hours later, the doctor found that not only was I fully dilated, but my baby was moving out of me. He smiled at my doula and said, "This is because of you." I was the talk of the hospital for days.

—Salma, 34, professor, mother of four

In fact, Dr. Friedman observed what he called a "deceleration phase" at the end of active labor, when it is to be expected that dilation will slow down. Today doctors are uncertain whether this exists; it may be that some mothers naturally decelerate while others do not. Especially with the use of Pitocin, it is not likely that deceleration would be noticed.

Penny Simkin, a respected founder of the doula movement, has brought attention to the following explanations for a seemingly stuck labor.

In the weeks before birth, some women go through a process of dilating as much as 3 to 5 centimeters without contractions. When a woman's labor actually does start, her provider may think she is already in active labor based on her dilation. However, she may only be in early labor, if her contractions have not yet increased in strength and frequency. She may not dilate quickly right away, and a doctor may incorrectly diagnose that "active" labor is stalling—when it really has not even begun.

Sometimes a buildup of lactic acid in the body can happen during birth, like with any athletic event, and this can temporarily slow labor, as reported by a study at the University of Liverpool in the April 2004 issue of the journal *Obstetrics & Gynecology*. Using Pitocin in these cases may only increase lactic acid. At these times, contractions may decrease simply because a woman's body needs to rest. Once lactic acid clears from the system, labor will usually naturally resume.

Finally, it is important to understand that lying down causes contractions and dilation to slow down. You can use this to your benefit if you are getting fatigued in labor, as lying down may allow you to rest or sleep when you need it. (However, a provider may not recognize this effect and may think labor is stalling in an abnormal way.)

A mother tells the following story:

> Near the end of labor, I felt sleepy and stressed, and I didn't know if I could keep going. My doula said, "Now is a good time to lie down and rest." It worked and I felt better. But because contractions slowed down, my doctor said I was "off the curve" and he wanted to use Pitocin. The nurse asked him to wait a half hour. Then I got out of bed, and I finished dilating on my own by the time the doctor came back.
>
> —Mary, 19, sales clerk, mother of one

## ᘓ LET GRAVITY HELP ᘔ

The strength of a contraction is rated in units known as *millimeters of mercury,* or mm Hg. (This is a way of measuring the amount of tension in the muscle.) When resting between contractions, the tension in the uterus is less than 15 mm Hg. Contractions that are strong enough to dilate the cervix need to be 30 to 50 mm Hg above the uterus at rest. And the strength of contractions increases by 35 mm Hg *simply by the mother being upright!*

When you feel the urge to start pushing, most providers have been taught to perform a vaginal exam to see if your cervix is completely dilated. You have the option of declining this exam (or any exams during pushing).

If the cervix is not fully open, providers typically ask mothers not to push. Their concern is that pushing against a cervix that is not completely open will cause damage to it. However, many women report that not pushing feels nearly impossible if the urge is present; anecdotal reports show that a woman's *natural* urges are unlikely to cause problems. (Simply avoid the forceful pushing of the Valsalva maneuver to protect the cervix.)

During pushing, providers may use vaginal exams more than at any other time in labor. These exams may help detect whether the baby has moved down, although this is not always accurate; also, by pushing on the inside of the vagina with one's fingers, the mother's stretch receptors respond by making her push. But remember the principle of removing disturbances during labor? Your body will push on its own without these exams.

Doctors commonly set deadlines for pushing, which vary depending on the provider or hospital. Most doctors will wait at least two hours, but some decide to perform a cesarean sooner than this for "failure to progress" during pushing, even if the baby is healthy and the mother may simply need more time to give birth.

Research in the *American Journal of Obstetrics & Gynecology* in October 2002 showed that it can safely take babies three hours to move just 1 centimeter during pushing (in order to descend to the mother's pubic bone); the study confirmed that most babies are born within a half hour after passing this landmark.

In medical terms, the dilation phase is known as the *first stage* of labor; the time from full dilation to the birth of the baby is known as *second stage,* and is said to consist mainly of pushing, although there can sometimes be extensive periods of rest during this phase.

The results of a nationwide survey were published in the

*Journal of Obstetric, Gynecologic, & Neonatal Nursing* in 2004; in this study, women pushed safely *for up to eight hours.* While the idea of pushing forcefully for that long sounds very unappealing, it is completely possible that a mother might not feel any urge to push until several hours after full dilation; then it could take several more hours for the baby's head to rotate, descend, and mold, and for the urge to build to full strength. Anecdotal reports from midwives, doulas, and mothers show that occasionally, a healthy second stage can take much longer, lasting as many as ten to twenty hours. Being patient and encouraging the mother to rest (not push forcefully) is the key to success during this phase.

## TWELVE ALTERNATIVES TO A VAGINAL EXAM

> In the usual context of modern birth, it is the midwife's or the doctor's finger that gives information about the progress of labor. When a woman is allowed to give birth according to the method of the mammals, the finger is uncalled for. Many aspects of the mother's behavior—her breathing, the noise she makes, her position—provide the attendant with much more insight.
>
> —Dr. Michel Odent, renowned obstetrician
> and author of eleven books

Whether or not you feel the need to limit vaginal exams, it is fascinating to realize they are not the only way to determine labor is moving along. Numerous signs of progress exist, some that a mother can observe herself, and others that involve alternate techniques used by the care provider. An experienced practitioner or doula can often estimate dilation using these techniques, *without* a pelvic exam. (When an exam is used, it often simply confirms the outward signs.) Some of these signs of progress are listed below; think of them as a reminder that dilation alone may not deserve the importance it has taken on.

### 1. CHANGES IN CONTRACTIONS
Contractions become stronger, longer, and closer together. Contractions two to three minutes apart usually correspond to active labor and dilation beyond about 4 centimeters.

### 2. THE HEIGHT OF THE BELLY
The top of the belly moves *upward* as labor progresses. At the beginning of labor, the space between the bra line and the top of the uterus is about the width of five fingers (during a contraction). Late in labor, this space is only about the width of one finger, corresponding with full dilation.

### 3. BLOODY SHOW
The appearance of blood-tinged vaginal discharge is a sign that the cervix is opening (as tiny blood vessels break during dilation).

### 4. "THE BOTTOM LINE"
When dilation is complete, a dark red or purple line that's about ten centimeters long can be observed in the crease between the woman's buttocks, as described by doctors writing in the medical journal the *Lancet* in the 1990s.

### 5. DESCENT OF THE BABY
Along with dilation, the baby gradually moves down in the mother's pelvis. Though this can be detected with a vaginal exam, the World Health Organization says it is more accurate for the provider to press the

outside of the mother's belly to feel for descent, known as external palpation.

### 6. THE BABY'S HEARTBEAT

As dilation increases, the provider will hear the baby's heartbeat in a lower location on the mother's belly. For a fun way to see progress, a pen can be used to mark the belly with an *X* each time the heartbeat moves lower.

### 7. BAG OF WATERS BREAKING

After contractions start, the bag of waters breaking on its own is a sign that labor is moving forward; it also usually indicates that labor will speed up from this point on.

### 8. ULTRASOUND

An ultrasound machine on the outside of the belly can be used to provide an image of the baby, to confirm descent, rotation of the head, and whether the baby is head down or in a breech position.

### 9. RECTAL PRESSURE

As it gets closer to the time to push, the mother will feel increasing pelvic or rectal pressure (like constipation) from the baby's head. The woman may grunt involuntarily. After 10 centimeters, her rectum will flare out.

### 10. INVOLUNTARILY HAVING A BOWEL MOVEMENT

This happens commonly during pushing. (Try not to worry; it's normally a tiny amount of stool, most laboring women don't notice, and your provider will clean you up as it happens.) It is usually one of the best signs the baby is really coming down and out.

### 11. "OPENING THE BACK"

During pushing, a small area above the mother's tail-bone bulges out, serving to enlarge the pelvis. According to anthropologist Sheila Kitzinger, Jamaican midwives say, "The baby will not be born until the mother opens her back."

### 12. SEEING THE HEAD

The baby's head will start to become visible at the opening of the vagina, indicating that dilation has reached 10 centimeters, the baby has moved down, and she'll soon be born.

### Another Point of View

Gloria Lemay is a doula trainer and traditional midwife, and was an advisory board member of the Canadian Doula Association. She reminds women they have the option of feeling their *own* cervix for dilation. She explains, "Your vagina is a lot like your nose—other people may do harm if they put fingers or instruments up there, but you have a greater sensitivity and will not do yourself any harm." Just as sexual touching is safe during pregnancy, so is this kind of self-exploration. Women who charted their fertility before pregnancy may already be familiar with touching their own cervix and feeling for its changes. (Refrain from inserting anything into the vagina if the waters have broken or there is heavy bleeding.) This is Lemay's description:

> The cervix in a pregnant woman feels like your
> lips puckered up into a kiss. When it is dilating, one
> finger slips into the middle of the cervix easily (just
> like you could slide your finger into your mouth eas-
> ily if you are puckered up for a kiss). As the dilation
> progresses the inside of that hole becomes more like
> a taut elastic band and by 5 cm dilated it is a perfect

rubbery circle like one of those mason jar rings that
you use for canning, and about that thick.

While this option may not be for everyone, numerous
women report getting to know their bodies in this way. This
is not meant to be a substitute for medical care, but rather a
way for women to discover their own anatomy, or as Lemay
would say, to reconnect with a sense of "ownership of their
bodies." Your cervix, after all, belongs to you!

## BEFORE YOUR WATER BREAKS, READ THIS

One scenario in which providers commonly use a timeline in
labor is when a woman's water breaks first, before contractions start. For the majority of mothers, their water does not
break until they are almost at the end of labor. But for about 8
percent of women, their water does break first. (On TV sit-
coms, the woman is usually doing something like sitting in a
restaurant when her water breaks, and everyone begins shriek-
ing and rushing to the hospital, but this is not what happens in
real life.)

Most doctors have been taught that a woman must begin
labor or birth her baby within twenty-four hours of her membranes breaking to lower the possibility of a serious infection.
If the water breaks first, many doctors tell their patients to
come to the hospital and begin an induction with Pitocin.
When twenty-four hours have passed, this time limit may be
used as a reason for a cesarean section.

While bad infections are very rare, they can cause serious
harm to babies; forty years ago, the search for a way to further
reduce their incidence was the logic behind this time limit. A
longer period of time with ruptured membranes is associated
with more infections. However, more current research shows
*the use of vaginal exams* is the primary factor that raises the risk
of infection; the passing of time has not been shown to be the
cause by itself.

In the early 1900s, a main cause of mothers dying in child-birth was contracting infections from doctors doing vaginal exams without washing their hands, because it wasn't under-stood that this transmitted germs. These infections were known as *childbed fever,* and the resulting death rate became epidemic in some European and American hospitals. The practice of hand-washing and the development of antibiotics were the greatest contributions medical doctors made to re-ducing deaths in childbirth, of which they had also unknow-ingly often been the cause.

Today, providers strictly follow *sterile technique* when con-ducting vaginal exams, which involves the use of a glove that has been completely covered in a protective seal. This reduces the chance of delivering germs from the room into the wom-an's vagina. But still, exams push bacteria that are *already* in the vagina upward and deposit them right onto the cervix with the provider's fingers.

Once the bag of waters has broken, the uterus is no longer protected, and the mother and baby can be infected. However, without a way for bacteria to travel upward, the flow of amni-otic fluid down and out of the woman's body continues to pro-tect them from infection.

Starting with the first vaginal exam, the chance of infec-tion rises with every exam. A major international research project known as the Term Prelabor Rupture of Membranes Study looked at risk factors for infection in more than five thousand women. With three vaginal exams, the risk of infec-tion doubled; with nine exams, the risk of infection soared five times higher. Scientists also conclude that risk of infection increases based on hours between the *first vaginal exam* and de-livery (not between *water breaking* and delivery).

Modern care providers would be wise to take a lesson from the days of the childbed fever epidemic. Countries such as Israel are strict about prohibiting exams after the water breaks, while U.S. providers tend to continue exams. The use of Pitocin to induce labor after the water breaks, and the use of cesareans after twenty-four hours, do reduce the number of infections somewhat. But these are dramatic measures to take when the elimination of vaginal exams most likely would have prevented the risk of infection in the first place.

Infections of the uterus can be caused by a wide variety of bacteria; the most common is Group B strep (GBS). Many women carry the bacteria in their vaginas, and the presence of GBS can come and go throughout pregnancy. Caregivers now test pregnant women for GBS close to the end of pregnancy to determine if it is likely to be present at birth. If GBS is present, providers give antibiotics in labor, which reduces transmission of the bacteria to the baby. However, *even the presence of GBS is a much lower risk factor* than having multiple vaginal exams in labor!

The World Health Organization says that infection might be caused by vaginal exams not only in labor but during prenatal appointments with your midwife or doctor; if you are GBS positive, you may want to avoid exams during pregnancy or inserting anything else into your vagina (e.g., use lovemaking options that don't involve penetration).

―――――――

If your water breaks before labor begins, what are your options?

Most doctors and midwives want to be notified when your water breaks. Your provider will probably ask you to come to the hospital to confirm this is what happened. Amazingly, many providers wish to use a vaginal exam to determine whether the bag of waters broke. Of course, this increases the chances of infection! However, you may request that tests for fluid be done outside your body.

Various tests can determine if your water broke, such as using a treated strip of paper to test the pH of the fluid, although the answers to these tests can sometimes be wrong.

False positive results can occur in the presence of blood, semen, antiseptic cleansers, or bacterial vaginosis. If you continue to feel and see periodic gushes of clear fluid, this is a good sign that it probably is your bag of waters.

Your provider also wants to check that the baby's umbilical cord did not slip out when your water broke. This is a rare scenario, but an unsafe one, and slightly more likely if the baby is breech, premature, or high up. Vaginal exams are sometimes used to check for the cord, but listening to the baby's heartbeat can reveal the condition of the cord instead.

The doctor will check for signs of infection, primarily a fever in the mother. Other signs can include a rapid heartbeat in mother or baby, foul-smelling vaginal discharge, or tenderness in the belly. The provider will see if the waters are clear, or stained with an old or new bowel movement by the baby; a new bowel movement may mean the baby needs to be watched more closely.

When there are no signs of infection or problems (which is most likely to be the case), some doctors and midwives will instruct women to go home. However, many doctors are trained to induce labor right away, to lower the chances that labor will take more than twenty-four hours.

If you are interested in the option of preventing infection by eliminating vaginal exams, rather than using Pitocin, you'll need to negotiate and ask clearly for this. If it is not your provider's standard approach to let labor start on its own, your request may be met with surprise or pressure to induce. But you probably will not have to wait that long for natural labor; according to the Cochrane Collaboration, 70 percent of women have contractions within twenty-four hours, 90 percent by forty-eight hours, and it can be safe for women who take longer if they're watched by their providers.

A variety of options exist for waiting for labor to begin:

- You may be allowed to return home and watch yourself for signs of infection, probably by taking your temperature every four hours to check for a fever developing.

- You may be allowed to return home with the arrangement that you come to the hospital every twelve hours, to check vital signs for you and your baby. This could mean you make numerous visits to the hospital over the course of several days; you may feel more pressured to induce labor each time you return. Also, you might find the idea of repeatedly going to the hospital to be an unwanted hassle. However, you'll be able to get plenty of rest between your twelve-hour visits, and it may be worthwhile to you to avoid a preventable induction or cesarean.

- You may have the option of checking in to the hospital and "living" there until labor starts. Your hospital may have *antenatal* rooms (used for pregnant women who are not in labor, such as those on bed rest). Or you may be admitted to an actual birthing room and allowed to wait; however, you may feel pressured to start an induction every time a provider comes in. (Debate exists about whether home or hospital is more likely to be a source of infection while awaiting labor.)

Two mothers had the following experiences:

My water broke before labor, and I was admitted to the hospital. After talking it over with my doula, I asked my doctor to wait until the next day to see if labor would start on its own, which she agreed to. This was not her usual way; she said that in ten years of being an OB, she never had the experience of seeing a woman wait more than twenty-four hours for labor to start.

—Crystal, 31, waitress, mother of two

My plan was to have my baby at a birth center outside the hospital, but my water broke when I was six months pregnant. I was checked in to the hospital and put on bed rest, in the hopes that labor *would not* start prematurely. An entire month went by there, which was a pretty unusual situation, and my doctor decided my bag of waters finally sealed up on its own. I was discharged from the hospital, and I went on to have my baby at the birth center with my doula at nine months.

—Collette, 44, school principal, mother of one

## ⤳ EPIDURAL FEVERS ⤳

It is important to be aware that one side effect of epidurals is an increased chance of fever. In most cases, *this* kind of fever is not caused by an infection, and is therefore not dangerous; it is believed that epidurals can cause fevers because of the way they act upon the nervous system. However, there is no way in labor to tell whether a fever is caused by an infection, or is simply the harmless side effect of the epidural.

Epidural fevers are treated as if an infection is present, on the small chance this may be the case, with antibiotics, Pitocin, timelines, and/or cesareans. It will take two days after the birth for lab cultures to tell if there had been an infection, or if it was just the epidural. Eliminating vaginal exams will not eliminate epidural fevers, because they are not related. But still, limiting exams may help reassure you that a fever with an *epidural* is less likely to mean there is a harmful infection.

## ARE VAGINAL EXAMS MEDICALLY NECESSARY?

Dilation checks alone have not been shown to detect medical problems, although they are routinely and widely practiced. Dr. Murray Enkin, obstetrician and longtime researcher for the Cochrane Collaboration, has commented: "Repeated vaginal examinations are an invasive intervention of as yet no proved value. Those who advocate its use have the responsibility to test their belief in an appropriately controlled trial." In select situations though, vaginal exams may provide medically necessary information.

If you are doing natural childbirth, there may be no need for vaginal exams as long as you and the baby are healthy. However, if you have an epidural, Pitocin, or other drugs to stimulate labor, vaginal exams become more medically relevant, as explained by Susan Cassel, CNM, former director of doula training for ALACE. Your provider may need to judge whether the drugs are affecting dilation, and whether the dosage of drugs is adequate for the desired effect, as well as safe. Even so, you can request that exams be done for the purpose of determining safety only; clearly ask how often exams are required, then remind your provider of the agreed-upon number of hours between each exam.

Once you are in active labor, the guidelines of the American College of Obstetricians and Gynecologists are for a caregiver to listen to your baby's heart rate once every fifteen to thirty minutes. If your provider feels unable to assess whether you are in active labor by using outward signs, she may request an exam in order to know whether to begin checking the baby's heart rate at this frequency.

During pushing, if the baby's head remains posterior or misaligned, a special technique may be used to help turn the baby. This technique is known as *digital* or *manual rotation.* Using a vaginal exam, the doctor or midwife places the tips of her fingers on the back of the baby's head, then guides it into the ideal position. By using this technique, in a pilot study in the March 2007 *European Journal of Obstetrics, Gynecology and Reproductive Biology,* the cesarean rate for malpositioned babies was reduced from 23 percent to zero.

In some cases, if the midwife or doctor determines labor may be proceeding unsafely and the baby needs to be born quickly, a vaginal exam may be needed to tell whether delivery is about to happen. These scenarios can include heavy bleeding in the mother, abnormal heart rates in the baby, or other problems. When vaginal exams are needed for emergencies, obviously your cooperation is important.

A mother tells the following story about the helpful use of a vaginal exam:

> Because of my personal beliefs, I chose not to participate in tests such as ultrasounds during my pregnancy. However, when I was in labor, my doctor thought my baby was unexpectedly breech. He did a vaginal exam and felt my daughter's bottom instead of her head, then he did an ultrasound which confirmed she was breech. The hospital staff was not prepared to deliver a breech vaginally, so I had a cesarean. Although things didn't go at all the way I planned, I was able to accept that the interventions were done because they were medically indicated.
>
> —Lilia, 36, opera singer, mother of one

> ### ◈ ASK YOUR DOCTOR NOW ◈
>
> If you are interested in the option of eliminating routine vaginal exams, start discussing this prenatally with your provider. What does he or she believe are medically urgent reasons to do exams? Is he familiar with using techniques other than pelvic exams to assess progress, like measuring the baby's descent by feeling the outside of your belly? If your water breaks and you show no signs of infection, would he support your waiting for labor to start on its own for one, two, three, or more days?

Since dilation checks do not reveal whether the baby is healthy, what procedures do provide that information?

In spite of the tremendous use of technology in today's births, doctors actually have few tools they can use to accurately detect emergencies in labor. Their most sophisticated technique is to listen to the baby's heartbeat with Doppler ultrasound or even a simple stethoscope, but there is not just one heart pattern linked to problems with the baby. Doctors disagree about how to interpret heart rates other than those that are perfect or terrible, leaving a wide range in between that are not well understood.

When a baby's heart rate seems worrisome, this has traditionally been described as fetal distress. However, the phrase "fetal distress" refers to the *possibility* that an infant is experiencing problems in labor, not the certainty of it. Most of the time, doctors are simply unable to clearly detect, or prevent, naturally occurring problems.

Although in a few cases a poor heart rate in the baby might be linked to cerebral palsy, according to *Williams Obstetrics* and the Cochrane Collaboration, 70 to 90 percent of the time when brain damage occurs in newborns it is not caused by events in labor and cannot be stopped by the birth provider. And while cesareans for fetal distress have increased, the rate of cerebral palsy has not changed, as reported in the *Journal of the American Medical Association*.

Scientists have determined that for monitoring of the baby's heart to be most useful, it should always be used with *fetal scalp blood sampling* if fetal distress is suspected. This procedure is mildly invasive to the baby; it involves placing a tube into the mother's vagina, and drawing blood from the baby while it is still inside the mother. The blood is then quickly analyzed in a lab to see if its pH is too acidic, which confirms that oxygen to the baby has been reduced.

Prenatally, you can ask your caregiver if fetal scalp blood sampling is offered at your hospital, and if so, request that it be used during labor if fetal distress is suspected. According to the Cochrane Collaboration, studies involving over 58,000 women show that "the increase in cesarean section rate is much greater when scalp pH estimates are not available."

## ∽ WHAT IS FETAL DISTRESS? ∼

### A GUIDE TO THE BABY'S HEART RATE

Doctors, midwives, and nurses look at several things when evaluating the baby's heart rate; it is not as simple as saying the baby's heartbeat is too high or too low. First, providers determine the baby's *baseline* (resting) heart rate. A full-term baby's normal baseline rate is 110 to 160 beats per minute.

Second, the provider looks for *variability* in the heart rate. This means that in the course of one minute, the baby's heart rate goes up and down; a change of more than five beats per minute is normal variability, while variability of less than five beats is cause for concern.

Third, the provider looks for changes in the heart rate known as *accelerations* and *decelerations*. An acceleration means the baby's heartbeat goes up during a contraction (and at other times, such as when the baby is awake and moving), and this is almost always considered "reassuring."

Decelerations refer to a decrease in the heart rate during contractions. Decelerations are caused by a wide range of events, some of which are a normal part of labor, such as pressure on the baby's head during pushing. However, other instances of decelerations, or "decels," may indicate a problem.

Regarding decelerations, *Williams Obstetrics* states, "the two most common causes are hypotension from epidural analgesia and uterine hyperactivity due to oxytocin stimulation." In other words, *epidurals and Pitocin cause the most decels—* the kind that are more likely to create anxiety in the delivery room.

Decelerations can also occur when the umbilical cord is squeezed by contractions in a way that may be fine for the baby, or may not be fine. They can be a result of the mother's prolonged breath-holding during pushing, or a serious problem with the placenta.

It is considered acceptable for the baby's heartbeat to go as low as seventy beats per minute before it is seen as worrisome, as long as this does not happen repeatedly or for long periods of time.

In the 1990s, the American College of Obstetricians and Gynecologists recommended that the term "fetal distress" be replaced with *nonreassuring fetal heart rate,* but clinicians have been slow to adopt this change in vocabulary.

When the baby's heart rate indicates possible distress, a number of treatments are used to restore it to normal. These remedies can be as simple as changing the mother's position, turning off Pitocin, using IV fluids or drugs to correct low blood pressure, or having the mother breathe normally instead of holding her breath during pushing. If the heart rate cannot be brought to a normal pattern, a cesarean is done.

In a 2007 study in the *American Journal of Obstetrics & Gynecology,* doctors identified at least 134 different patterns that a baby's heart rate can take on in labor! These patterns include many possible combinations of fast or slow heartbeats, high or low variability, and decelerations that come early or late during a contraction. Most of these patterns fall somewhere in between excellent and horrible. And *at least 50 percent of babies* have a heart rate pattern somewhere in that middle ground. Using the baby's heart rate to determine whether it is healthy is the best tool we have, yet it is highly imprecise and open to interpretation.

## HOW TO HAVE A GREAT PITOCIN EXPERIENCE

When it looks like Pitocin is in your future, and waiting for labor to take its natural course is not an option, how can you make the best of this situation?

First, if your provider wishes to schedule a date to *induce* labor with Pitocin (or other drugs), you may consider these options as an alternative:

- Staying sexually active, by yourself or with your partner, may make it unnecessary to have an induction. According to the journal *Obstetrics & Gynecology,* women who had sexual intercourse an average of four times in the ninth month of pregnancy gave birth sooner and were half as likely to be induced as women who did not have sex. (But you needn't consider sex to be a requirement if it is physically or psychologically uncomfortable, or not acceptable for cultural or religious reasons.)

- The Cochrane Collaboration reports that breast stimulation is as successful as Pitocin for starting labor within three days. Tell your provider before you use this method, as it might cause contractions that are too strong in mothers who are "high risk." (However, studies show contractions from breast stimulation are generally less strong than with Pitocin.) You are most likely to get results using an electric breast pump one hour per day. Each time you get a contraction, *stop breast stimulation* for five minutes before starting again, to mimic natural labor. Also, stop completely if you have contractions longer than one minute each. You can also consider this technique if your water has broken without contractions, or if labor is under way and your provider wants to use Pitocin to speed things up.

If it's been decided that Pitocin definitely will be used, keep these tips in mind in order to have a healthier and happier experience:

- You can use all the labor support techniques you normally would: massage, staying out of bed, walking, etc. You may even be allowed to take a shower or bath for pain relief.
- Request a low dose of Pitocin that is increased more slowly. This may be all that is needed for the desired effect; providers refer to this as a "whiff" of Pitocin. (It's delivered by IV, not by breathing in a whiff of it.) Studies also show this is safer than a high-dose regimen that is increased more rapidly.
- Turn to your loved ones, your doula, or your provider for a pep talk. Focus on the positive aspects of the experience: "The baby is still healthy, we're in this together as a family, it's normal to need a few minutes to feel upset about a change in plans, you can have your other wishes met (remind yourself what they

are), you're doing a great job, let's still have fun with this!"

- Pitocin requires constant monitoring of the baby's heart. Ask for a portable wireless monitor so that you can continue to stay active and leave your room for a walk down the hall.

- Once contractions are two to three minutes apart ask to have Pitocin turned off, because your body may continue to produce frequent contractions on its own.

- Watch for extremely long contractions that go on for more than ninety seconds each, or contractions that seem to have only a tiny break of a few seconds between them. Pitocin needs to be turned down or off in these situations for safety, and although providers should be checking on this, studies and doulas report that they don't always notice.

- When women need pain medicine to cope with Pitocin, they usually choose an epidural. However, some women use the option of IV narcotics instead. Even though contractions with Pitocin can be stronger than natural labor, and narcotics give less pain relief than epidurals, some women choose narcotics because they prefer not to have an epidural. (Narcotics need to be used before pushing, so they are not in the baby's system at birth.)

- If you need an epidural after receiving Pitocin, get a "walking" epidural. (See chapter 4 for more information on its benefits.)

- Pitocin can lead to an epidural, or an epidural can lead to Pitocin. Epidurals can slow labor, but they sometimes have the opposite effect; by allowing muscles to relax, sometimes dilation increases rapidly with an epidural. Ask to see if this happens before going right to Pitocin.

- Getting into a tub of warm water may also speed dilation, and may allow you to skip Pitocin altogether. A study in the *British Medical Journal* showed that when women with "stalled" labors got into a tub for up to four hours, one in three mothers who would have gotten Pitocin didn't have to.

- If you and your baby are healthy, ask your midwife or doctor to give Pitocin the time it needs to work. According to scholar and doula Henci Goer, research shows that women who are given only two hours on Pitocin to achieve increased dilation receive three times as many cesareans, compared to women allowed to continue laboring for four hours or longer with Pitocin.

Remember, you are still giving birth to your baby. It takes courage to give birth whether interventions are used or not. When Pitocin is used, it is not because your body "just wouldn't open up the way it was supposed to." Do not fault yourself if your hospital has a timeline or if health problems require that the baby be born more quickly. Give yourself credit for all the amazing work you do in labor, Pitocin or not!

Although there is currently a heavy emphasis on dilation, vaginal exams, and timelines for giving birth, labor is not about dilation. Your body knows how to give birth whether or not you ever have a pelvic exam in labor. Birthing women need encouragement to trust their bodies, and to be the stars of their own labors. Doulas help provide this encouragement. And the confidence a woman discovers in labor can help carry her through the demands of parenting and future challenges in life.

# 9

# LABOR TECHNIQUES ANYONE CAN USE

Most labor techniques require no special expertise, or even any practice. Comfort techniques can be very effective, yet amidst the overwhelm of labor and the distractions of a typical hospital, these techniques are often abandoned or forgotten. What makes a technique work isn't mastery of complicated methods. Women in normal labor mainly need to feel a sense of security, permission, and sometimes gentle, steady persuasion to put these techniques to use so they can have an effect. (When practice is involved, it is practice in the sense of trying something out ahead of time, not becoming an expert at it.)

According to the "Listening to Mothers" survey, the labor techniques mothers report as the most helpful are never actually tried by the majority of women. These include actions as simple as getting out of bed to relieve pain and boredom, something anyone can do (unless she has a disability—see the upcoming sidebar). So, what's wrong with this picture?

As it turns out, the necessary encouragement is not so easy to find in hospitals, many of which are understaffed. Studies show that nurses need to spend 90 percent of their time on medical procedures and note-taking, with little left over for labor support.

Doulas are in the perfect role to keep track of all the possible comfort measures, and to guide you in techniques appropriate for many different scenarios as you climb the mountain of labor. A doula is there to notice, "How do *you* give birth?" She strives to make sure you're helped in labor as an individual, without assuming the same procedures and techniques should be used on every woman.

Following are the labor techniques reported by mothers, doulas, and research to be the most effective.

### Freedom of Positioning

The most basic technique known to speed labor, decrease pain, and reduce the use of medical interventions is to simply get out of bed. Yet over 75 percent of U.S. women report that after they are admitted to the hospital, they never leave their beds. Why? Several factors probably influence this: television images tend to portray women laboring in bed; lying down is the position caregivers are most familiar with; and moving a nine-months-pregnant woman in labor takes a little more effort than you might think.

However, changing positions is one of the most important labor techniques and offers many benefits. Some positions are less painful than others, and freedom of movement allows a woman to discover which positions work best for *her*. Upright positions are better than horizontal ones in most cases, because contraction strength or *uterine pressure* is significantly increased, and the cervix dilates faster.

Upright positions can be more beneficial for the baby's heart rate, because the mother's blood pressure is less likely to drop, and because the weight of the heavy uterus is not lying on major blood vessels in the mother's back. And women who walk in labor report fewer cesareans, according to surveys conducted by Childbirth Connection.

Positions in which the belly hangs forward are often helpful, including facing and leaning on a support person, or leaning on furniture. These positions move the baby away from the mother's back and can prevent the extra pain of back labor. Also during contractions, the uterus normally tilts itself forward (away from the mother's back). If the mother is leaning forward, her uterus can easily and naturally tilt forward, too. But if the mother is lying back, her uterus must work harder to tilt forward, therefore causing more pain.

Lying down and staring up at caregivers or even at loved ones can sometimes produce feelings of helplessness, compared to the psychological benefits of sitting totally upright or being in other vertical positions.

Changing positions in bed while pregnant is not the easiest thing, as you may know from turning over in bed at home. Surprisingly, sometimes providers are reluctant to help move a woman even a small amount, such as from her back to a fully side-lying position, or from reclining to fully upright, because it takes physical effort from the caregiver to assist, or they are skeptical that it will make a difference. You may need to insist on help with changing positions. (Hospital staff are better trained to move a patient's weight *safely;* loved ones need to be careful not to injure themselves when doing so.) Even a position shift of a few inches may make more room in the pelvis for the baby to come down, or significantly relieve pain.

The positions and movement options available are many, including standing, walking, climbing stairs, swaying, lunging, sitting, crouching or squatting, leaning forward, being on hands and knees, kneeling, and side-lying.

## ⌬ DISABILITIES ⌬

A woman may have a physical disability or chronic medical condition that affects her mobility; usually she is the person who is most knowledgeable about the capabilities of her own body, and she can share this information with her doula and obstetric caregivers in order to receive the support she needs to have the most positive birth experience.

Disabilities can include spinal cord injuries, joint conditions such as rheumatoid arthritis, conditions involving bone malformations, conditions affecting the muscles such as muscular dystrophy, and numerous others. They may be accompanied by symptoms including numbness, paralysis, joint or soft tissue pain, limited range of motion, stiffness, the ability to walk only a limited distance, or muscle weakness.

As a woman with a disability, you are probably well aware of which positions are feasible for you and which are not. For example, you may require pillows under your joints when you are lying down in order to diminish pain related to the disability, or lying on your back may simply not be an option for you. If you know that sitting with your back supported or lying on your side work well, for instance, clearly let your providers know, and return to your favored positions regularly.

## ᘯ DISABILITIES ᘰ

(continued from previous page)

According to Judith Rogers, author of *The Disabled Woman's Guide to Pregnancy and Birth*, tools that may be available to assist you in positioning yourself include: the incline controls on a hospital bed, a raised toilet seat or cushions to raise the seats of chairs, a footstool to use when sitting, and a shower chair. Be sure to ask for help locating these items so you are not unnecessarily limited by not having access to them.

Depending on your physical capabilities, many of the positions we've discussed may be beneficial to your labor, including being on hands and knees, sitting completely upright, or side-lying. Squatting may be possible with the use of a "squatting bar" to hold on to, available at many hospitals. Ask the staff to physically assist you in position changes, and take as much time as you need to experiment or make adjustments until you are comfortable.

Throughout history, women in a role similar to that of doulas spent much of their time physically holding up the laboring mother. The anthropologist Sheila Kitzinger notes that this type of support has been observed in locations as diverse as Jamaica, Japan, Peru, Thailand, and West Africa. She comments:

> It is not merely a matter of "positions" for delivery, but of providing physical support for movement

during contractions. Movement is facilitated when a woman has another human body to hold or lean against, or when she is grasped in strong arms by a helper who is alert to respond at the onset of each contraction, providing a firm stationary base or moving in unison with her.

This type of constant physical assistance is largely unavailable from hospital staff, but it can be achieved with the use of a doula, a willing spouse, or other labor companions who understand that supporting a birthing woman can be hard physical work for the helpers, but a highly effective technique for labor.

## ෴ YOUR ROOMY PELVIS ෴

While you're still pregnant, you can get to know your pelvis, and have more of an understanding of the benefits of being able to position your body so your baby can move through it.

Try this: Press your fingers into the creases at the tops of your inner thighs, near your groin area. Press firmly until you feel the two bones of your pelvis on either side. Your baby will be coming out of your vagina in the space between these bones. With your fingers in place, move your hips from side to side, then rotate your hips in a circle. Next try walking, then crouching.

Notice how the space between the bones (and your fingers) widens as you move. The change in dimensions may seem small, but it is just enough to help when your baby is passing through. These changes of a few centimeters are what are so important in labor!

## Emotional Techniques

Above all, labor is an experience of personal vulnerability and transformation. As such, birth is accompanied by powerful emotional, psychological, and spiritual needs. Awareness of your own emotions, and the sensitivity of those around you, will be vital to helping you through.

A variety of approaches exist for addressing the emotions of labor, including visualization, hypnosis, prayer, and mind-body techniques. We will be focusing here on ways to simply ask yourself what it is you are feeling, and how to express those feelings and share them with others.

During labor, find times to check in with your feelings. You can do this quietly and alone, although it is also helpful to share your emotions with your loved ones. And when possible, try to share your feelings honestly with your doctor, midwife, or nurse. Studies show that rates of interventions such as cesareans may be lower, and mothers rate their births more positively, when caregivers are aware of the emotional needs of their patients.

### GET IN TOUCH WITH ☜ YOUR EMOTIONS ☞

Following are questions you can ask yourself in the midst of labor. (You can also ask yourself most of these questions while you are still pregnant; pregnancy is a time of emotional sensitivity, and your need to get in touch with your feelings may already be strong.) The most basic way to check in with your feelings in labor is to ask yourself these kinds of questions:

- Do you feel good about what is happening now?
- What is your intuition telling you?
- What is it you are afraid of?

Your doula might also ask questions to help you get in touch with your emotions, such as:

- What would make this a great birth experience for you?
- What do you need from your loved ones in the room?
- What do you need from your doctor/nurse/ midwife?
- How do you feel about becoming a mother?
- How do you feel about the baby?
- How do you feel about pushing your baby out?
- How do you feel about feeding your baby?
- Are you thinking about your own mother right now?

The following questions may also be helpful during labor, if they apply to your situation:

- How do you feel about your previous birth(s)?
- If you are having a vaginal birth after cesarean, what are you feeling about it?
- If you are deciding whether or not to use pain drugs, do you have worries about this decision?
- If your provider is recommending a medical procedure, what feelings are you having about it?

Emotional techniques involve not only feeling your emotions, but expressing them in a way that feels helpful to you. In labor, you'll probably be able to answer most of the questions above by simply talking about them. It is also OK to cry out, swear, moan, yell, weep, or otherwise vent your emotions during birth, if this helps you feel a sense of release. However, if your emotions are spiraling into panic or terror, ask for help becoming more calm; this is different from the "normal" stress of labor. (Also, if reading these questions while you are pregnant brings up strong negative feelings, we encourage you to discuss them with a counselor before you are in labor.)

Many women try too hard *not* to vent their emotions in labor, or worry about being unkind to those around them. If you feel inhibited about how you'll behave in labor, you can practice ahead of time by moaning, groaning, and giving yourself permission to let it out—try this in the shower! Labor will be easier if you are free to express yourself, rather than struggling to keep it together. (In some countries it may be considered culturally unacceptable to make noise in labor, but other forms of coping may be available instead, such as biting on a rolled cloth.)

Family members can give emotional support by saying loving things and asking the birthing woman how she is managing. When loved ones witness the intensity of labor for the first time, they are sometimes unsure about what to say to the mother. It is appropriate to use simple phrases of encouragement that feel natural, such as:

- I love you.
- You're doing a great job.
- How are your spirits?

### Warm Showers, Baths, and Jacuzzis for Pain Relief

Showers and baths serve a different purpose in labor than in everyday life. The point here is not to get in, wash up, and quickly get out, but rather to use warm water as a form of pain relief, which can be dramatic. The Cochrane Collaboration reports substantially less use of epidurals and less pain in women who labor in water. Mothers who use baths and showers rate this as the most effective method of non-drug pain relief. And yet only 10 percent of American mothers ever try this technique.

Warm water promotes relaxation by increasing circulation and lowering blood pressure, by stimulating the skin on your entire body (like a water "massage"), and in the case of baths, by providing buoyancy which takes strain off the heavy uterus and belly. To reap the full effects, make your showers and baths in labor *long,* especially at the hospital, where there is plenty of hot water. For the most pain relief, it is recommended that you stay in for up to ninety minutes at a time!

In *active* labor, studies show that use of a bath can help speed up labor. However, baths in *early* labor can slow things down. Also, after about ninety minutes in a bath, a shift in hormone levels can occur, and labor may slow down. Therefore, when you are ready to take a break from the bath, get out for thirty minutes to balance this effect. You can get in and out of water as many times as you like in labor.

If interventions such as Pitocin, an IV, or constant monitoring of the baby's heart are required during birth, you may still be able to get into water. Many hospitals have some portable waterproof equipment, although it may take extra time to locate it; be sure to request this from your providers in labor. (In the case of an epidural, getting into water is currently not an option.)

Using a bath in labor does not mean you are required to have a water birth, where the baby is actually born in water. The option of *laboring* in water has become more widely available in hospitals, but the option of water birth is still less available. When available, underwater birth can be a wonderful option for some mothers; for more information about what this experience is like, see the Web site of Waterbirth International at www.waterbirth.org.

If you normally enjoy using very hot water, be aware that baths in pregnancy and labor should not be heated to more than one hundred degrees Fahrenheit (thirty-seven degrees Celsius), for the baby's safety. Get a bathtub thermometer at the drugstore to use for baths at home if you are not sure what your water temperature is.

In hospitals, showers are found more commonly than tubs or Jacuzzis. When tubs are available in hospitals, they are usually the size of a standard home bathtub. A few hospitals as well as alternative birth centers offer larger tubs; the benefits of a larger tub are that a partner can sit in the tub with you for closeness, and the tub may be deeper, allowing your entire belly to be submerged underwater for increased pain relief.

When using a tub in labor, fill the water as high as possible in order to cover your pregnant belly. Even a few additional inches of water can make a difference, so don't stop at a shallow amount of water. It is possible that reclining in a tub may not be comfortable (just like reclining in bed can be uncomfortable in labor). If this is the case, don't abandon the tub; simply shift so you are sitting completely upright in it. In a larger tub, you can turn onto your hands and knees, or kneel while resting your arms over the side of the tub.

### Touch and Massage

Touch and massage have been used throughout the ages during birth. Most women love being touched in labor, when it is done in a way that is sensitive to their needs. On rare occasions, a woman truly does not wish to receive any touch in labor, and she ultimately knows what's best for her. But in most cases, touch can be tremendously comforting, pain-relieving, and relaxing.

Mothers who use touch and massage rate it the second-most effective natural pain relief method. Yet 80 percent of women report never actually trying it in labor. As with some other techniques, you probably will not be able to rely on hospital staff to provide touch and massage in labor. One study looked at 616 interactions between nurses and laboring women; nurturing touch occurred only 2 times.

Benefits of touch include increased levels of the hormone oxytocin, which speeds labor and promotes a sense of well-being. (Synthetic Pitocin does not produce the effect of well-being because it is delivered through the bloodstream by IV, rather than being manufactured in the brain like natural oxytocin.) Studies from the Touch Research Institute at the University of Miami show that women receiving massage in labor report less pain, less anxiety, and have shorter births.

According to doula researchers Dr. Kennell and the Klauses, fathers-to-be touch their partners about 20 percent of the time in labor, while doulas touch mothers up to 95 percent of the time. However, the exception to this is when both the father and a doula are present; in these cases, the amount of time fathers touch their partners is *increased.*

Touch from partners can take many forms, including: hugging, holding the mother's hand, stroking her hair, kissing her, sexual touching when privacy is available, wiping her face or neck with a wet washcloth, cuddling, sleeping next to her in the hospital bed, or massage.

The use of touch can be as simple as a support person placing his fingers on a part of the mother's body that looks tense and gently saying, "Relax your forehead," or "Relax your shoulders." This can be repeated over and over in labor, until the mother remembers to release these areas of tension on her own.

A doula tells the following story:

> Labor is work, and it builds up heat in a mother's body. At some point, I usually wipe a woman's sweating brow with a washcloth. After I did this at one birth, her partner went right over, climbed in bed with her, and began the same motion of wiping

her forehead. It wasn't something I told her to do, but I could see she felt it was OK to try it after watching me. I was happy my presence helped this partner feel confident about staying close to the laboring mom. And without trying, I had demonstrated something she could easily do to bring her relief.

Is massage really something anyone can do? Yes! Although professional massage therapists have developed hundreds of strokes to use on all areas of the body, almost all massage techniques come down to two basic motions: *caressing* and *squeezing*.

## CARESSING

A caress is a kind of touch that is loving and caring. It works best when the motions are slow rather than fast. Make contact with your entire hand and palm. (You can also caress with your fingertips, but this can create more of a poking effect than a soothing one, so be sure to ask the receiver of the massage how it feels.) Caressing does not take a lot of strength to do, and should not be tiring for the giver; try to keep it going for ten to thirty minutes, or until the receiver is ready for a break. Caressing can be done during contractions as well as between them.

Caressing can be done anywhere a "line" is formed on the body: all the way down the arms, down the legs, down the whole back, or along the sides of the face. Caressing can also be done in circles on larger areas: caress in a big circle on the back, or in a large circle on the pregnant belly (do this lightly, and avoid the woman's belly button, which can be sensitive).

Caressing can be done over the mother's clothing or on her bare skin. To give a massage you can use your bare hands, or coat your hands with a simple moisturizer like lotion or vegetable oil from the kitchen. (Professional massage oil is simply a blend of various vegetable oils.)

SQUEEZING

To try squeezing techniques, start by standing behind the mother and giving her a shoulder rub. Again, make contact with your whole palm, not just your fingertips. Grasp the muscles at the top of the shoulders and squeeze with a medium pressure. Ask the receiver if she wants less pressure or more. Squeezing takes more strength than caressing, so you will probably only do it for about five minutes at a time.

Use slow motions with squeezing too, rather than fast ones. Other places to squeeze include the back of the neck, the upper arms, the muscles around the lower back, the front and back of the thighs, the hands, and the feet. Squeezing is for smaller areas, while caressing is for longer lines of the body.

Squeezing should be done between contractions (not during them, when the stronger pressure may feel irritating to the receiver). There is an exception to this, known as *counterpressure.*

COUNTERPRESSURE

Counterpressure involves pressing firmly on certain areas to give relief during contractions. One area to press is the *sacrum,* the spot on a woman's back that is below her waist and above her tailbone. Inside the body, the sacrum is where the uterus is attached to bone, and women often feel a strong ache here during contractions. When a support person presses this area, a mother often feels relief. Use the palm of your hand or your knuckles to press her sacrum. This is also one of the most important techniques to use for the pain of back labor.

Another technique to use during contractions is the *double hip squeeze,* made popular by doula leader Penny Simkin. The support person stands behind the mother, and firmly presses his hands into the muscles of her buttocks on both sides. This results in a sense of release for the pregnant woman, and can greatly relieve pain across her entire abdomen. It takes a lot of strength from the support person, so do this for only about one minute at a time. Or do it with two helpers, so that one person presses into the mother's buttocks from each side.

Most forms of touch do not require practice in advance; you can easily hug a woman in labor at any time. However, mothers who are partnered can "practice" cuddling during pregnancy, and all mothers can try out massage with their support person ahead of time. The mother and the support person can take turns being the giver and receiver. This way the mother can show the support person how strong she likes the pressure of a massage to be. Don't be shy about asking for loving touch when it is needed, or about giving it!

### Eating Normally in Labor

The option of eating in labor has been debated and largely banned in American hospitals for decades. The reason is not that eating is bad for labor, but that years ago, eating seemed to pose a danger if general anesthesia was used during birth. In the 1940s, Dr. Curtis Mendelson published research showing mothers might vomit under general anesthesia and then choke, a problem known as *aspiration*. Bans on eating in labor followed.

However, general anesthesia is rarely used in today's obstetrics, and medical techniques to prevent aspiration have greatly improved, making the mortality rate of this complication extremely low. The U.K. Department of Public Health reports that it occurs in one in two million births, even with eating being more commonly allowed in British hospitals than in the U.S. Other countries freely permit eating in labor, without showing an increase in negative effects. Nonetheless, these bans are still mostly in place in U.S. hospitals. (Alternative birth centers and home birth providers tend to encourage eating.)

The main benefit to eating in labor may simply be that women feel less miserable when they are not starving, according to research published in *Ob.Gyn. News* in 2007. Therefore, staying nourished becomes a coping technique for labor.

(Studies show mixed results as to whether eating improves other outcomes, such as length of labor and rates of interventions.) It is estimated that women need at least fifty to one hundred calories an hour to meet the demands of labor, a physically strenuous event. Because a typical first labor can last twenty-four to forty-eight hours or longer, the discomfort of not being allowed to eat can be significant.

How can a mother best negotiate with her hospital about the option of eating? When women ask for permission to eat, hospital staff often simply reply that it is not allowed. Some hospitals are more permissive of eating as long as drugs have not been administered, but others are strict about prohibiting food even during natural childbirth. Once medications are in use, especially epidurals, this is the point after which eating (and sometimes drinking) is nearly universally forbidden in U.S. hospitals. At this point in labor, fluids are given by IV so that dehydration is not a concern, but calories and nutrition are not available.

Trying to negotiate in the midst of labor about the right to eat can be stressful. It may be better to discuss your wishes with your midwife or doctor prenatally instead. You can bring research to discuss with your provider, such as "Restricting Oral Fluid and Food Intake During Labor" from www.cochrane.org, or "Providing Oral Nutrition to Women in Labor" from the American College of Nurse-Midwives, at www.jmwh.com. These conversations can help inform caregivers about an outdated practice, and even if they are not ready to make a change in protocol, it lets providers know patients want these options to be available.

If you have a medical condition that could be negatively affected by a lack of eating or low blood sugar, such as epilepsy or type 1 diabetes, you can also ask to meet with an anesthesiologist at your hospital prenatally, as this is the person who often has the most influence over whether nourishment is allowed. You may or may not need to use pain drugs during your actual birth, but you can ask the anesthesiologist to recommend that you be permitted to eat more liberally in labor, and to put her recommendations in writing.

When you are in labor, whether to eat is ultimately your personal choice, even though the hospital staff may strongly discourage or wish to prohibit it. Do your best to avoid a heated confrontation about this provocative issue, while knowing that you do have the right to choose to eat normally.

It is helpful to bring your own food, since the hospital cafeteria may have limited hours of operation. A laboring woman as well as her loved ones need to keep track of staying fed; labor will only be getting more intense and demanding of everyone's stamina! Pack nonperishable energy food in your bags ahead of time, such as raisins, nuts, dried fruit, granola, nutrition bars, and sports drinks. Studies show that hunger levels vary among individual women during birth. As labor unfolds, follow your own body's cues about whether or not *you* need to eat.

## HOW TO SLEEP IN LABOR

Did you know that sleeping during childbirth is possible? Not only that, but when faced with the immense forces of labor, preventing the extra strain of sleep deprivation is one of the most important things you will need to do. Think of it as another essential labor-coping technique.

In the midst of labor, here's a good way to remind yourself of the importance of getting enough sleep. Unless you are almost finished dilating or you're pushing, ask yourself the following question periodically: "How will I feel if I am still in labor twenty-four hours from now?"

For example, when labor starts you may be filled with excitement, and sleep may not seem that important, or even possible. Let's say labor starts around dinnertime, and you find yourself eagerly staying up past bedtime, wondering if things are about to kick into gear, even though contractions are still ten minutes apart.

Although it might be two AM and you don't have the urgent desire to sleep, ask yourself: "How will I feel in twenty-four hours?" In fact, you may not even *begin* active labor for another twenty-four hours. You'll want to have as much sleep under your belt as possible when you finally get there.

Dr. Gayle Peterson, an author and expert in the psychology of pregnancy and birth, makes the following observation:

> Some women stop eating or sleeping because they are excited and believe themselves to be in labor. They are, of course, but usually it is only early labor. What I call the beached-whale syndrome occurs when a woman uses up all her resources early in her labor. She doesn't get the sleep, rest, or food that she needs, resulting in total exhaustion by the time she reaches the active phase. By then she may be so depleted she requires medical intervention.

Do what you can not to let that scenario happen to you! It is a common mistake, and an understandable one. However, remember that early labor with a first baby almost always necessitates that you try to sleep at some point, despite the excitement and physical discomfort you may feel.

### How to Sleep in Early Labor: At Home

LIE DOWN IN A DARK ROOM, even if you are too excited to fall asleep right away. It is important to at least let your body rest, in a horizontal position in the dark, for as long as possible during overnight hours. Also, lying down results in less frequent contractions.

TAKE A WARM BATH, which can slow or temporarily stop the contractions of early labor (but not advanced labor) so you can rest, according to the *Journal of Nurse-Midwifery*. A bath may also encourage drowsiness. You may need to stay in for a full ninety minutes for contractions to stop.

YOU MAY DRINK A GLASS OF WINE to help you to fall asleep. Besides helping you feel drowsy, alcohol is considered a *tocolytic,* or labor inhibitor, and may give you a couple of hours without contractions. (Historically, doctors gave it to mothers by IV to stop premature labors.) If you'd like to consider this option but don't normally keep wine at home, remember to get a bottle well before your due date.

CONSIDER SLEEPING IN A SEPARATE BED from your partner if you're both restless, so he or she will be less preoccupied with labor having started, and less likely to become sleep-deprived, too.

DRINK EXTRA FLUIDS AND WATER. An early labor that is not strongly established will often slow down and allow you to rest if you maintain good hydration.

### How to Sleep in Advanced Labor: In the Hospital

CREATE DARKNESS AND QUIET in your room, and play soft relaxation music. (You'll probably need to bring your own portable stereo.) Ask your doctor or midwife and nurse to allow you to rest without coming in and out of your room for one or two hours.

A PARTNER OR DOULA CAN PROVIDE CARESSING to help mothers relax and lull them to sleep. Of course, it will not be like normal sleep once labor is well established. But many women are able to doze between contractions, then wake during contractions, and doze again between. Mothers can gain up to several hours of sleep this way.

YOU MAY BE ABLE TO REQUEST MEDICATION to induce what is known as *therapeutic sleep,* usually with a one-time injection of a high dose of morphine. If labor is still mild, the effects may last long enough to gain almost a full night of sleep.

LOVED ONES, TAKE A NAP IN THE HOSPITAL. The birthing woman needs you to stay rested and save your stamina for the end of labor, too! A doula can help massage the mother to sleep, while her partner naps for an hour or two on a hospital cot. After the partner naps, he or she can trade places with the labor assistant. Bring earplugs and a sleep mask to fall asleep more easily in a busy hospital environment.

## LABOR TECHNIQUES
## ANYONE CAN USE

### BRING THIS LIST TO YOUR BIRTH!

**TO THE MOTHER IN LABOR**

- To keep contractions strong, **stay upright** (stand, sit, walk, kneel, squat).

- Take **long showers or baths** for pain relief (up to ninety minutes, if possible).

- To relieve **back pain,** get onto your hands and knees.

- Ask for a **portable heart monitor** for the baby, so you can move freely and leave your room.

- Share your **emotions and fears** with your loved ones and providers.

- **Make sounds,** sigh, moan, and let yourself cry when needed.

- During overnight hours, **lie down in the dark,** to slow contractions and rest.

- **Eat** to provide at least fifty to one hundred calories an hour.

- If you need anesthesia, ask for a **low-dose epidural** and help with position changes.

- **While pushing, remain upright** (stand, kneel, squat, sit on the toilet) or use a side-lying position for more effective results.

**TO HER LOVED ONES**

- **Give the mother reminders** to use the above techniques.

- Being careful not to strain yourself, **physically assist her to change positions,** or ask the staff to help.

- If there is room, **get into the shower or tub** with her for closeness.

- **Slowly caress** the mother's arms, legs, back, and face.

- **Squeeze** her shoulders, back of the neck, thighs, hands, and feet.

- **Say encouraging things** and ask questions such as:

    "I love you."

    "You're doing a great job."

    "How are your spirits?"

    "What would make this a great birth for you?"

- Make sure that **you eat and sleep.** Ask, "How will we feel if labor is still going on twenty-four hours from now?"

*From* The Doula Guide to Birth *by Lowe and Zimmerman. May be copied for individual use.*

# 10

# When Epidurals and Cesareans Are Unplanned

*I was under the impression that planning for
natural childbirth would prevent a cesarean section.
But for me and some of my friends, it didn't, and that
came as a difficult surprise.*

—Linda, 33, social worker, mother of one

*The most important thing I learned when I was
working as a nurse-midwife at an obstetric ward was
that every mother wants to have a special, wonderful
childbirth experience. This is true even though birth
itself is of diverse and mostly uncontrollable processes.*

—Rieko Kishi, advocate of doulas in Japan

Mothers who hope for natural childbirth, and then achieve it, usually report high satisfaction with their births. Similarly, when a woman plans to have an epidural and then does so, or a cesarean is scheduled in advance for medical reasons, studies show her chances are also good for feeling positive after her birth.

However, when a mother plans to avoid these interventions, or simply does not expect them, but finds they must be used, her chances of feeling negative about her birth are increased. According to the book *The VBAC Companion* by Diana Korte, women who experience an unplanned cesarean are at highest risk; these moms report up to six times the rate of depression postpartum. Fathers and partners may also be affected.

"Planning" for the unexpected sounds like an oxymoron, but it is a necessary undertaking for all pregnant women: whether you intend to have natural childbirth, an epidural, a home birth, or a scheduled cesarean.

Mothers who desire natural childbirth have the highest chance of achieving it at home, where 90 percent do so. About 80 percent of those using alternative birth centers have natural childbirth. (Women in both of these settings still need to have a plan B for how they would cope with being transferred to a hospital.) In the U.S., approximately 80 percent of mothers birthing in hospitals have epidurals, and over 30 percent undergo cesareans; the use of a doula can reduce these rates by about half, but even those who use doulas have a chance of encountering interventions, simply because they are considered routine by most hospital staff.

Women's feelings of satisfaction, disappointment, and even trauma after birth have been researched in countries as diverse as Australia, Belgium, China, France, Saudi Arabia, the U.K., and the U.S. In spite of the availability of this research, women's emotions about their births, including depression, are not always acknowledged by their caregivers. A 2004 report presented at the University of California, San Francisco shows that health-care workers view birth experiences differently than mothers themselves, with providers often viewing cesareans more favorably than their patients do.

These studies from around the world are in agreement about the factors that determine whether a mother sees her birth as positive, negative, or traumatic. The most important factors are:

1. Whether a woman's expectations of birth match the reality of what happens
2. Whether a woman feels involved in decisions about her care, even if her expectations cannot be met

Although birth is naturally accompanied by a sense of vulnerability, this is different from a sense of helplessness. Studies show that when women evaluate their births, even the pain of labor is less important than whether they felt helpless about their options.

Based on these findings, scientists from Belgium concluded in 2007, "the empowerment of laboring women, not the management of childbirth by means of painkillers, leads to satisfactory birth experiences." Thirty years earlier, Dr. Murray Enkin of the Cochrane Collaboration commented on the importance of involving mothers in their own care: "The decision to perform a cesarean section is one which the physician can make. The decision to have a cesarean birth is one which the parents should make."

Not only are women's birth memories affected, but research shows that even lawsuits against caregivers are influenced by whether mothers feel included in decision-making.

## HOW CAREGIVERS
### ᗡᔕ CAN LISTEN ᔕᗡ

Fairly or not, sometimes patients and doulas must help "teach" caregivers how to meet the mother's needs. In labor, one of the best ways to do this is to express your emotions honestly in front of your providers. This includes any possible negative feelings about an unplanned epidural or cesarean. When caregivers are aware that a woman feels afraid, disappointed, or conflicted, they may be better able to respond humanely to her feelings.

## HOW CAREGIVERS
### ෴ CAN LISTEN ෴

*(continued from previous page)*

Tekoa King, the nurse-midwife who presented the report at UC San Francisco, proposes the following guidelines for health-care workers. Before leaving a patient's room or proceeding with an intervention, a caregiver should ask himself:

1) How does his behavior acknowledge the mother's expectations?

2) Does the mother feel safe and in control following her interaction with him?

Why might an unplanned epidural or cesarean affect a mother's emotions so strongly? For one thing, preparing for birth is like preparing for other events of great personal magnitude, such as planning a wedding or a trip around the world, except birth is filled with even more intensity. These kinds of events carry the potential for bliss as much as for despair. Sue Radosti, a doula and trauma therapist, comments:

> Childbirth is an experience of unrivaled vulnerability, encompassing all that is most personal and most precious: a woman's physical safety, her sexuality and body image, her beliefs and values, her deepest emotions and attachments, and her hopes for the future.

Physically too, interventions are invasive to the body. Especially when they are unexpected, a woman may feel overwhelmed by these physical intrusions. Epidurals and cesareans involve the insertion of needles, drawing blood, the use of a catheter in the bladder, and sometimes other bodily procedures; in the case of cesareans, of course, cutting is involved. The hurriedness of these procedures may result in stress for the mother followed by longer term psychological injury.

Back at home with an infant (or multiples), mothers are emotionally vulnerable as they adjust to their new roles and responsibilities. Especially if they do not have enough support postpartum, some women feel they are unable to come to terms with a difficult birth; in this unresolved state, they struggle to concentrate on the needs and demands of a newborn, and bonding may be affected.

Physically, cesareans can interfere with a mother's ability to carry and respond quickly to her baby. With epidurals and cesareans, breast milk may be delayed in coming in, and other side effects can impact nursing. These physical effects can contribute to depression. In fact, a potential risk of any surgery is depression, yet providers often forget to inform cesarean mothers to watch for this.

Although these scenarios may seem daunting, it is possible to be better prepared for surprises, and to find the inner and outer resources to deal with them more positively should they occur. Birth and parenting always require courage and strength. For a mother who encounters unplanned birth interventions and difficulties, the opportunity for discovering inner strength and healing can also be available to her.

## "PLANNING" FOR THE UNEXPECTED

We encourage you to think ahead of time about the needs you might have in case of an unplanned epidural or cesarean. Be reassured, imagining the unexpected doesn't cause it to happen. (Nor does it prevent it.) But if you do find yourself in labor faced with the unexpected, you'll benefit from having prepared for it.

> I chose a home birth for my baby, which was a
> careful and important decision. Most of my labor
> did take place at home, with the support of my

midwife and doula, my boyfriend, and my two sisters. But near the end, an old back injury of mine acted up and made it too difficult to cope with everything. We agreed to go to the hospital for an epidural.

This was definitely different from what I was hoping for. But during my pregnancy, my boyfriend and I tried to imagine this possibility. Our daughter was born easily and shortly after we got to the hospital. When we found ourselves in the midst of unwanted events, I was more at peace because we'd done our best to picture them in advance.

—Olga, 35, boutique owner, mother of one

While you are still pregnant, take the time to imagine yourself facing the following situations. These are scenarios in which birth interventions are unplanned, but ultimately a decision is made to use them. (There may be other situations in which an intervention is suggested and the mother declines it, but for the purpose of this chapter we are addressing interventions that do get used.)

Discuss each imaginary scene with your partner or support person and with your doula. Don't shortchange this conversation; you'll probably need a good hour for it. (Doulas should also contemplate these questions, and their own feelings about them.)

You may experience discomfort as you partake in this exercise; if so, recall the words of Dr. Gayle Peterson, an authority in the psychology of pregnancy and birth:

Acknowledging fear can deepen our reserves and help us discover fresh meaning and commitment in our lives. Do not judge your fear or anxiety. Confront and befriend the fear, and it will yield an inner treasure.

Ask yourself these questions:

1. Imagine that an epidural is necessary during your birth. What feelings do you think would arise for you?
2. If an epidural is needed, what would help make this the best possible scenario for you?
3. Now imagine that a cesarean is necessary. What emotions do you think would arise?
4. If a cesarean is needed, what would help make this the best possible situation for you?
5. What fears or anxieties do you have about these situations? (Be sure to give them a voice before your actual birth.)
6. How have you (and your partner) responded to unexpected stress at other times in life?
7. What would you want your doula, and your doctor or midwife, to remember about your needs in case of unplanned events during birth?

## YOU STILL HAVE OPTIONS

Even when labor diverges from an ideal image, a range of options may still be available to you, and knowing you have choices can help you to remain empowered and feel positively about your birth.

Here are some points to keep in mind if an epidural is needed. You will have more options for a variety of positions in labor if you can request a low-dose epidural. (This is also known as a "walking" epidural, although it may not be possible to literally walk. See chapter 4 for more information.) The best remedy for many of the drawbacks of an epidural is to *change the mother's position.*

When epidurals lead to side effects, a mother often feels more stress. It is possible to take steps to minimize these risks. Side effects can include a drop in the mother's blood pressure, which may result in one or more episodes of fetal distress, or labor may slow down and lead to the use of Pitocin or a cesarean for "failure to progress." The use of completely upright positions is an easy and effective technique to help prevent these situations, and can be done with an epidural.

The use of forceps or a vacuum to pull out the baby is more common with an epidural, if pushing seems to be going slowly. Surveys conducted by Childbirth Connection show that more than 90 percent of U.S. mothers are instructed to lie on their backs or recline during pushing. Only 4 percent push on their sides; yet side-lying may result in more successful pushing, according to New Zealand midwifery expert Jean Sutton.

Other options with an epidural include turning the epidural down (or even off) if you would like to feel more sensation again. Also, remember to continue incorporating labor support techniques after an epidural, especially massage. Some women report they no longer received enough emotional and physical support after an epidural. With massage, the giver should avoid squeezing areas of the body that are numb; however, caressing and loving touch are still appropriate on areas that are not anesthetized. Touch also produces natural oxytocin, which may help avoid the use of Pitocin after an epidural.

With an epidural in place, you may want to use this quieter time for spiritual reflection, or to talk or think about labor or the baby. Loved ones, remember that although the mother is attached to monitors that may draw your attention, the machines are not having the baby, she is. Some people choose to turn on the TV with an epidural, but be sure to give the birthing woman the attention she still deserves.

---

How can a cesarean be more empowering? In the case of a true emergency, it may not be possible to avoid rushing, along with the stress that accompanies it. In this case, strategies for emotional recovery may be especially needed postpartum, which we will discuss shortly.

If a cesarean (or an epidural) does not need to happen instantly, some women benefit from taking the time in labor to think about, discuss, and process the decision. For example, you might want to request fifteen minutes alone with your family and doula, or you may want an entire hour. You may want your provider to take additional time to explain the need for the procedure, its benefits and risks, and details about how it will be performed, so you feel you are participating in a more informed decision. You may also want extra reassurance that the baby is still healthy, and a pep talk to help you keep going in good spirits.

An unplanned epidural or cesarean *requires a psychological adjustment* to what is happening in the moment. It is normal to possibly feel confused, upset, or to feel a sense of loss about what was hoped for. Feelings of disappointment or fear may be surprisingly strong. If possible, go ahead and take time to let these emotions out, including crying if needed. There is often relief in expressing emotions rather than holding them back, so you can participate in the rest of your birth more fully.

On the other hand, it feels more natural for some women to begin their medical procedures without delay. These mothers may feel more empowered moving forward quickly once a decision has been made, rather than waiting and engaging in longer discussions. If you find yourself facing interventions, ask for as much or as little time as you need, based on what suits you best.

The environment for a cesarean resembles what you'd think an operating room looks like: lights are bright and the OR is generally lacking in "softness." Not much can be done to change this, but you may have some choices about the *sounds* in the room. There might be a portable stereo available, or you can ask to bring your own, along with music to help comfort you. There's some truth to those TV shows that depict doctors talking about golf or politics during surgery. This distraction may feel comfortable for some mothers, but others may want to ask for more quiet. Some women like to have a staff person describe the surgery as it happens, while others prefer not to hear the details.

Right after the cesarean, a caregiver will take the baby to an examining table in the room, which may or may not be within the mother's view. Many women intensely wish to know what is happening with their baby at this moment. Unless there is a dire emergency, it is usually fine for the woman's mate or support person to talk lovingly to the baby, and to describe to the mother what the baby looks like if she wishes. This can be enormously comforting to her.

Remember to bring your camera into the operating room! Most hospitals allow photos to be taken of the baby, and occasionally of the surgery or the moment of birth. The woman's partner or doula can be the photographer, or there might be an unoccupied staff person who can do so. If a mother wants these types of photos, they can be comforting for her to look at in the future when she is trying to recall the sequence of unexpected events.

After being examined, the baby will be shown to the mother while the surgery is being repaired. She might have the freedom to hug her baby on her chest, or someone may hold the baby near her. After a few minutes, it is the protocol in many hospitals for a caregiver to take the baby to the nursery, even if he is healthy, because the mother cannot "do" much while surgery is being completed. However, some families strongly prefer to avoid this separation. They can try to request that an exception be made, and the baby be allowed to stay with the mother for the entire surgery.

In the rare case that general anesthesia is needed for a cesarean, the mother will experience unconsciousness, and loved ones are not included in the operating room. A doula would remain with the family in a waiting room, and she can provide needed support during this time. A mother who has general anesthesia can ask for her medical records later, which can help her form a picture of moments that she missed out on.

## AFTER THE BIRTH

Following an unplanned epidural, cesarean, or other surprise events, a mother may experience several possible responses, including satisfaction, grief, or even trauma. If a woman's response to her birth is a negative one, her postpartum adjustment will also include the need for emotional recovery. Many women are left on their own to figure out this healing process, but we'd like to offer suggested guidelines, as well as to encourage these moms to turn to support groups and professional help when needed.

One of the most common emotions reported by women after unplanned interventions, unfortunately, is guilt. One mother described her experience this way:

> When I made the decision to have an epidural, the conflicts that went through my mind were not about any possible medical risks. All I worried about in that moment was whether I had "failed."
>
> —Susan, 34, interior designer, mother of one

Many women are confronted with these feelings, especially if they worked hard to prepare for getting through labor without drugs. As for cesarean section, a study from Sweden found that one in four mothers who had the surgery blamed themselves for needing it.

Why are feelings of guilt so prevalent? Part of the answer lies in the larger health-care climate in which mothers are giving birth. Natural childbirth has not received enough support in hospitals to be a real choice for all women who desire it. In this context, epidurals and cesareans do not feel like a completely free choice, either. Natural birth can become idealized, and interventions can be unfairly seen as a personal failure.

There is another reason why women sometimes blame themselves. Among the symptoms of grief or trauma, feelings of guilt are a normal part of these processes. (See the upcoming sidebar.) It is human to seek explanations after a loss; and oftentimes, we place responsibility upon ourselves. Women and mothers in today's society may be especially vulnerable to this kind of self-blame.

Try to remember that while feelings of guilt may be a normal coping mechanism, you deserve to let yourself off the hook, and to let go of finding yourself at fault.

Also remember that various scenarios involve abnormal levels of pain in labor, and that it would be inhumane to deny pain relief to someone experiencing them. These situations might include the use of Pitocin, back labor that does not go away, extreme nausea, and not having slept in days. The normal pain of labor is likely to be the most intense sensation a woman has ever felt, and is a fully legitimate reason in itself to choose medication.

As for a cesarean section, whether it is needed due to a medical problem or because today's intervention rates are unavoidably high, it is never the mother's fault when it occurs.

———————

*Grief* is the result of undergoing a loss. In the case of unplanned interventions, this refers to the loss of an experience that was hoped for. Many women report that if they express disappointment about an epidural or cesarean, their loved ones and caregivers have replied by saying, "You have a healthy baby, that's what really matters." (Of course, when a baby is not born in good health, a family is likely to experience increased stress.) But a woman's dreams about how she will birth are also valid, and should not have to be at odds with her hopes of safety for her baby.

To underscore this point, in 2008 the journal *Midwifery Today* hosted a seminar with doula leader Penny Simkin titled "There's More to Birth Than Coming Out Alive." A woman's feelings of dignity, emotional security, and her need to experience birth as the celebration of a major life passage are also important. When these aspects of birthing are compromised, her confidence about functioning as a new mother can be weakened.

*Trauma* is defined as a response of extreme fear, helplessness, and distress in the face of an event that is perceived as dangerous to the person having the experience. Post-traumatic stress disorder (PTSD) after a difficult birth is gaining attention as a condition that affects as many as 7 to 18 percent of new mothers, according to sources including doula pioneer Paulina Perez and Childbirth Connection. "Emergency cesarean" is the term often given to a surgical birth, and because cesareans are associated with potential emergencies, women who experience surgery are more susceptible to a possible trauma reaction.

## GRIEF AND TRAUMA
## ∞ SYMPTOMS ∞

Grief and trauma may have similar symptoms. Some women experience these emotions in response to unexpected interventions (or other difficulties, such as when a baby is not born in good health). Grief is a response to loss and may be accompanied by intense sadness, while trauma is a response to danger and may be accompanied by intense fear or anxiety. Either grief or trauma may include the following:

- Emotional numbness or shock
- Difficulty concentrating or making decisions
- Feeling emotionally exhausted or drained
- Blame toward others or yourself; feelings of guilt

## GRIEF AND TRAUMA
### SYMPTOMS

*(continued from previous page)*

- Replaying what happened in your mind over and over
- Urgently trying to figure out what could have been done to prevent what happened
- Feelings of aloneness
- Anger or irritability
- Loss of appetite
- Difficulty sleeping or sleeping too much
- Avoiding reminders of the birth, such as avoiding driving past the hospital where it took place
- Going through actions mechanically
- Feelings of detachment from the baby

## IF HEALING IS NEEDED

Emotional recovery is the process of returning to a more positive state after a loss. Some mothers feel disappointment after an unexpected epidural or cesarean, but adjust to it more easily, especially if they felt included and supported in decisions about their care. For others, the demands of caring for a newborn allow them to set aside their feelings about giving birth, and eventually they find that any negativity fades away on its own. However, many women need an outlet to express their feelings about what happened, and if one is not available, they may find that negative emotions become prolonged.

## SIGNS OF EMOTIONAL
## ~~ RECOVERY ~~

Just like grief and trauma consist of a collection of symptoms, recovery consists of a number of feelings and signs that things are getting better. These can include:

- A sense of aliveness rather than numbness
- An improved ability to concentrate
- Relief from feelings of despair
- A reduction of intrusive thoughts about "what went wrong"
- Accepting that you are not to blame
- A sense of connectedness to your baby and loved ones
- Relief from insomnia
- A return of normal appetite
- The ability to focus on the present and the future
- The ability to enjoy yourself again

The following approaches can be helpful when trying to make peace with unexpected interventions. You may have time to make use of these approaches shortly after birth, or you might find you are in need of them months or even years later. Ways to assist with healing include the following:

1. SPEAK TO A COUNSELOR OR THERAPIST, especially if you feel sad most of the time, or suspect you may be depressed or traumatized. You may even be able to find a counselor who specializes in issues of pregnancy,

birth, and postpartum by asking your caregiver or your doula for a referral. In the U.S., the National Association of Perinatal Social Workers can help you locate a specialist, at www.napsw.org.

2. CONTACT ORGANIZATIONS THAT OFFER SUPPORT after a difficult birth. The International Cesarean Awareness Network can be visited at www.ican-online.org. Birth advocate Sheila Kitzinger founded the Birth Crisis Network, at www.sheilakitzinger.com/Birth Crisis.htm.

3. WRITE YOUR BIRTH STORY. Allow yourself to express any and all feelings that come to mind. Think of this as being for your own eyes, not as a memento that you will save to show your child someday. You might choose to share it with your partner or a counselor if you wish to ask for their support, but this is not required.

4. SHARE YOUR STORY WITH OTHER MOMS who have had a similar experience. Compassionate discussions can be found on Web sites such as www.BabyCenter.com. For example, one mother recently posted the question, "How do I deal with my disappointment over having a cesarean?" This was followed by dozens of sympathetic responses from other mothers offering a range of viewpoints.

5. TALK WITH YOUR DOULA, YOUR MIDWIFE, or doctor about what happened at your birth. They may be able to supply helpful information about moments in labor you do not remember. You might also have criticisms you want to share. If you are not sure they would be understanding of your point of view, you may choose

to write them a letter instead. Think of the letter as a place where you can express any emotions freely, not necessarily as one that you plan to send.

In her book *An Easier Childbirth,* author and psychologist Gayle Peterson suggests numerous exercises to help resolve feelings after an unsatisfying birth experience. One technique is to create a visualization for yourself in which you imagine the birth you wanted to have, and to allow yourself to enjoy the imaginary experience. Especially for mothers who were separated from their babies due to a difficult birth, Dr. Peterson feels it can be soothing to conjure up feelings they may have missed out on.

Grief specialist Sherokee Ilse recommends that mothers make time to remember what was positive about their births, and to appreciate the ways in which their bodies worked well for them. This can include things like going into labor on your own, your bag of waters breaking on its own, getting through the beginning of labor, getting through many hours or days of labor, or growing a baby inside of you for many months.

Be aware that friends and family may not know how to talk about your birth in ways that are helpful. Mothers who experience interventions find that loved ones may focus on asking them, "What went wrong?" These moms may have the need to discuss this very question, but they also have the need to celebrate the births of their babies. If possible, clearly tell your loved ones what *you* need, whether it is their support as you grieve, or focusing on what is wonderful about the birth of your child.

Also, ask for extra help with breastfeeding. All mothers deserve more support for breastfeeding than what is generally available; epidurals and cesareans may increase the chances of difficulty with getting nursing started. Milk can be delayed from coming in, and babies' behavior can be more disorganized for several weeks. For women who had unwanted interventions, the wish to "succeed" at breastfeeding sometimes feels more urgent.

More hospital staff are now trained to help with breast-feeding, but sometimes this causes confusion in itself; that is, every person who interacts with you may offer different advice. Ask to see the same nurse or lactation counselor every day that you are in the hospital. Before you go home, ask the hospital staff for the name of a lactation support person whom you can call every day if needed. Early breastfeeding can benefit from *daily* support until it is more securely established.

When it comes to unplanned interventions, open communication is one of your greatest tools, from airing fears in advance of your birth, to making sense of the incredible event after it happens—and even helping create changes that will benefit families in the future, by letting others know what mothers really need.

> During my pregnancy, our baby's body was in a transverse position (sideways), which I learned is very rare. My doula helped me prepare for a regular delivery, and she also said we should discuss my emotions about a potential cesarean. I wanted to see if my baby would turn and I waited to go into labor naturally.
>
> My baby stayed in such an unusual position that a vaginal birth wouldn't have been possible, so I had a cesarean when labor started. I felt supported each step of the way during my pregnancy and birth. The cesarean happened safely, and it was ultimately a really positive experience for me and my family.
>
> —Loretta, 39, homemaker, mother of two

Finally, we'd like to introduce the idea of a *self-evaluation scale* that can be used by any woman after her birth, whether she feels her experience was positive or negative. A variety of scales have been developed over the last several decades to help mothers and researchers understand how women view their births. We have created an evaluation that appears as an appendix at the end of this book, and which you can use to help identify your feelings, including areas of satisfaction as well as possible areas of concern. Once you have filled out the scale, you can also share it with your caregiver, your doula, or a counselor as a way to begin a conversation about your needs for follow-up after labor.

## CONCLUSION

Whatever way birth happens, it is your rite of passage into motherhood, and that passage is to be celebrated. Natural childbirth is a passage, cesarean birth is a passage, and birth with an epidural is a passage to be celebrated. That passage cannot be taken away from you. Every mother's birth experience is valid, and an act of courage.

Sometimes it seems as though natural childbirth is idealized, because women have had to fight for the right to experience it. On the other hand, some women choose epidurals and cesareans gladly. Some women have these interventions under emergency conditions, while others feel pressured into them unnecessarily. The mothers in all of these situations deserve to have their births and their courage celebrated.

Pregnancy, birth, parenthood, and life are filled with dreams as well as losses. Do not hold back from celebrating the dreams come true, or grieving the losses from the bottom of your heart. And remember that with birth, sometimes it is necessary to do both at once.

# II

# BIRTH PLANS AND BIRTH ESSAYS

The use of birth plans and birth essays is a recent phenomenon. Both are documents that you can write to help communicate your needs to your caregivers, though they are used in different ways. The idea of a birth *plan* has received more attention, and we will be going into detail about how to create and use one. The birth *essay* is a lesser known but exciting tool that we will also be introducing here.

## THE BIRTH PLAN

Doulas helped invent the idea of birth plans; Penny Simkin was the first person to publish a brochure with guidelines for writing one in 1980. Today the concept is commonplace, and labor assistants frequently ask their clients to prepare a birth plan.

A written birth plan allows a woman to explain her requests for labor, including such things as comfort tools she would especially like to use, like a warm tub, and activities or procedures she might prefer to avoid, for instance frequent vaginal exams. These are only examples, as every mother's personal priorities will vary. Over the years, many people have designed detailed checklists of maternity-care choices to help women create their plans. We have designed a checklist for this purpose too, which appears later in this chapter.

We've placed this chapter near the end of our book so you would first have the opportunity to learn about some of the most central issues in labor and delivery today. Our birth plan checklist addresses topics thoroughly discussed in previous chapters, such as timelines in labor, pushing, and epidurals. And as Simkin has commented, a checklist reflects the bias of the people who designed it; this includes ours, as well. Birth plan guidelines have been created by everyone from activists for childbirth reform to mainstream hospital administrators, and the choices on these lists vary accordingly.

Your plan will reflect the issues that are most important to you. Our checklist does not include every possible scenario that might occur. However, there may be additional issues that you care about, due to your previous births, stories you have heard from other women, health conditions you might have, or other books you have read. If so, you can by all means include these topics in your personal birth plan.

In our book we've mentioned, but not discussed at great length, some of the birthing options and debates that have already been analyzed in other widely available books; these include such issues as inducing labor artificially, episiotomy, continuous electronic fetal monitoring, and home birth. For examples of checklists that address topics beyond the scope of our book, visit Web sites such as www.birthplan.com, or see Dr. Marsden Wagner's 2006 book, *Creating Your Birth Plan.*

In addition to medical procedures, birth plans can encompass a wide range of needs of the birthing family. Use your birth plan in whatever way is most meaningful to *you.* Birth plans can include anything from whom you would like to announce the sex of the baby, to the use of complementary health-care techniques such as acupuncture, to requesting a moment of silence when the baby is born so you can say a religious blessing.

––––––––––

When mothers present these documents to their obstetric caregivers, what response do they receive? While we encourage the use of birth plans, it's important to note they have sometimes garnered mixed reviews from hospital staff and birth advocates alike. Part of the reason is that labor, of course, cannot literally be planned. If a woman has strong expectations attached to her birth plan, she may suffer from disappointment if those expectations cannot be met, as we discussed in the last chapter. But ideally, birth plans can be used as a communication tool, helping caregivers be more aware of a mother's dreams for her birth, and guiding them to support her even if those dreams cannot be perfectly fulfilled.

## INTRODUCING THE
## ❧ HALF-PAGE BIRTH PLAN ❧

While checklists to help *prepare* a birth plan can be lengthy and detailed, going on for many pages, we believe the *final* written plan should be as short as possible. When mothers write very long birth plans, their caregivers may respond more defensively. After all, as a professional, no one enjoys feeling she's being told how to do every aspect of her job. Try to pick and choose the priorities that are truly most important to you, in the range of just a half-dozen wishes. (A half page may be all that you need, although it might not always be possible to keep it that short.) Numerous providers have replied to the briefest birth plans with a sigh of relief and enthusiasm, making it easier for them to say, "Now this we can help you with!"

Does putting their requests in writing increase the chances that women's wishes will be followed? One of the only studies on this topic appeared in a 2007 issue of the *Journal of Reproductive Medicine*. While this study was fairly small, it provided some insights into the most common desires expressed by mothers. In this study, 69 percent of women's birth plans stated they hoped to avoid pain drugs, but about half of them changed their minds in labor. Even so, women with birth plans were more likely to avoid epidurals than women without birth plans. Written plans did not seem to lower the rate of some other procedures, including cesareans.

It's been observed that a birth plan should not be used as a substitute for having trust in your provider. In response to the study mentioned above, obstetrician Marjorie Greenfield, the author of *Dr. Spock's Pregnancy Guide,* notes:

> With the exception of epidural use, doctors tend to manage labor the same way regardless of patient preferences. If you have preferences, you are better off choosing a team whose normal practices support your desires than creating a document to try to influence medical management.

Indeed, the most important factor in what type of birth you are likely to have is not whether you write a birth plan or take childbirth classes; it is knowing the standard routines of your caregiver and birth facility. We still feel birth plans are important, but it is also essential to inquire with your provider about the rates of various procedures they use, including rates of natural birth, epidurals, VBACs, and cesareans, to see if their approach matches your own.

For this reason, some mothers choose to interview several providers early on, or even to switch providers in the middle or late stages of their pregnancy. For other women, though, this step may not seem like an option for them. Their insurance may not cover another caregiver who interests them. They may feel too emotionally attached to their current provider to consider a change. Or they may find that every hospital in their area has an epidural rate of 80 to 90 percent, for example, and switching might not seem to make a difference. But within the same hospital, it is sometimes possible to find another caregiver (or group) that offers a different approach, and this may be worth investigating.

## ☙ KNOW YOUR HOSPITAL ☙

In addition to preparing your birth plan, know the trends at your hospital. The Transparency in Ma-

ternity Care Project was launched in 2006 to collect information on mothers' experiences with
caregivers and hospitals, to obtain official statistics on obstetric interventions at hospitals, and to
make this information available to the general
public. The project began in the U.S. and has plans
to expand internationally. To search for information about your provider or hospital, or to share
your experience, visit www.theBirthSurvey.com.

While a birth plan cannot control everything that happens, there are certainly advantages to writing one. This is
because in many hospitals, it is standard for doctors, nurses,
and midwives to care for two or more mothers in labor at the
same time. A written plan can distinguish you and your wishes
from those of several other women birthing on the same day.
Also, when caregivers change shifts, your birth plan can cue
them to remind the next provider of your requests.

## HOW TO CREATE AND USE YOUR BIRTH PLAN

It is helpful to start by writing a sentence or two that includes
personal information about yourself, giving the reader a flavor
for who you are. For example, you might want to mention
what kind of work you do, whether you've ever witnessed a
birth live, what happened during your previous births, or
whether you've had experience with other major physical
events, like running a long race. The readers of your plan will
be your caregivers, some of whom will be meeting you for the
first time in labor, and sharing personal information can help
them bond with you a little more quickly.

You can also use the opening of your birth plan to describe your overall approach to birth. For many women, one
of the most important questions to answer is: "How do you

wish to handle the potential pain or sensations of labor?" This is a highly personal question, and each woman's response will be unique to her. We'll be offering suggested ways to address this in our checklist, but we strongly encourage you to answer this question in your own words as much as possible.

Then you can use our checklist (or other checklists elsewhere) to select topics to include in your plan. Use part of your birth plan to describe your hopes as they relate to normal labor, if nothing unexpected happens. Also be sure to *include your wishes in the event of unexpected circumstances,* such as a cesarean section, or a labor at home or in a birth center that needs to be transferred to the hospital.

Write or type your wishes onto a new sheet of paper. This will be the first draft of your plan. Discuss it with your doula, and bring a copy to a prenatal appointment with your midwife or doctor. Be sure to ask your provider to give you feedback about each item on your list. If your provider is part of a group, you can ask if she thinks the other providers will be supportive of your plan. After having these conversations, you can revise your plan as needed, and make your final copy.

Once you've done this, you should not assume your provider will memorize everything on your plan; give her a copy and ask her to leave it in your health-care chart. You'll also want your birth plan to be available during your actual labor. Do not assume the copy you give your provider prenatally will be delivered to your birth; bring copies with you in labor. And finally, do not assume your providers understand everything exactly as you meant it. You may have stated something that needs clarification, they might misinterpret what you've written, or you might even have a typo. Ask for time to discuss your plan again upon arriving at your birth facility in labor and each time caregivers change shifts. Have your doula make sure that each doctor, midwife, and nurse who is caring for you takes a look at your plan.

## ✺ BIRTH PLAN CHECKLIST ✺

**INSTRUCTIONS**

Fill in the blanks on this list, and check the items that are more important to you. You may also want to consider other birthing options that are not on this list. We then suggest you narrow down your list to approximately five or six priorities, and rewrite just those items on a new sheet of paper to give to your caregivers.

Your name: _____

**YOUR SUPPORT PEOPLE**

(It is helpful to identify the support people at your birth, stating their names and relationship to you. E.g., your husband, wife, boyfriend, partner, baby's father, baby's adoptive parents, your mother, your sister, your other children, sperm donor father, friend, doula, etc.)

Name: _____ Relationship: _____
Name: _____ Relationship: _____
Name: _____ Relationship: _____

Personal information (about your job, your previous births, your approach to birth, or other topics of your choosing):

_____
_____
_____
_____

**PAIN RELIEF**

How do you wish to handle the potential pain or sensations of labor? *(Use your own words as much as possible to answer this question. Some suggested phrases appear below.)*

_____
_____
_____
_____

___ I would like to do natural childbirth; please do not offer pain drugs.

___ I prefer not to use the word *pain*. I would like to use words such as *sensations* or *surges* instead.

___ I wish to delay the use of pain drugs as long as possible.

___ I am open to natural childbirth or pain drugs and would like to decide this in labor.

___ I plan to use pain drugs, and I prefer (circle): an epidural/IV narcotics/other drugs available in this facility or country.

**LABOR TECHNIQUES**

___ If limited rooms are available with a tub, I would like to request one.

___ Please encourage me to use baths or showers for pain relief.

___ I welcome comforting touch and massage from my (circle): loved ones/nurse/midwife/doctor/doula.

___ Please encourage me to use upright positions such as standing, walking, leaning forward, kneeling, etc.

___ I have taken HypnoBirthing® classes and would like to use techniques such as: reading relaxation scripts, listening to CDs from the program, etc.

___ I prefer conversation and distractions in the room to be kept to a minimum.

___ I am familiar with belly-dance movements and would like to use them for pain relief.

VAGINAL EXAMS

___ I prefer no vaginal exams, except in case of a medical emergency.

___ I prefer vaginal exams only at these times (circle): upon arriving at the hospital/if I am trying to decide whether to use pain drugs/ to judge the effects of medication/at my request/other: _____.

___ If vaginal exams are done, I (circle) do/do not wish to learn how many centimeters dilated my cervix is.

___ I am agreeable to vaginal exams as my provider judges them necessary.

___ If my water breaks before contractions begin, please confirm this by testing on the outside of my vagina, not with a vaginal exam.

THE PACE OF LABOR

___ If my water breaks before contractions begin, I would like to wait for labor to begin on its own, even if longer than twenty-four hours, as long as my baby and I are healthy.

___ If labor is going slowly, I would like to labor without Pitocin, even if longer than twenty-four hours, as long as my baby and I are healthy.

___ If labor needs to start or speed up for medical reasons, I would like to try the following techniques (circle): breast pump/getting into a warm tub for ninety minutes/using an epidural without Pitocin right away/using Pitocin for at least four hours before a cesarean.

___ If Pitocin is needed, please use a low dose that is increased slowly, rather than a high dose that is increased more rapidly.

___ I am agreeable to the use of drugs such as Pitocin to stimulate labor as my provider judges necessary.

___ For safety reasons, I want to avoid use of the drug Cytotec (misoprostol), which has not been approved by its manufacturer for use on women in labor.

### PUSHING

___ I would like my caregiver to coach me in pushing. *(This is often the Valsalva maneuver or pushing with added force, along with the mother lying on her back.)*

___ Please, no loud coaching to "push."

___ I prefer a silent atmosphere during pushing.

___ I am interested in "laboring down the baby" without adding extra force to my pushing.

___ I prefer not to start pushing when I am first fully dilated. I would like to wait two hours or until the urge to push is overwhelming.

___ I prefer no vaginal exams or pressing inside my vagina by my caregivers during pushing.

___ Please encourage me to push in an upright position, such as squatting, being on hands and knees, or standing, not lying on my back.

___ If I am not able to be upright, please encourage me to push on my side, not lying on my back.

BABY'S HEART RATE

___ If I must remain on a fetal heart monitor continuously, please provide a portable wireless monitor so I can walk around.

___ If there are questions about the baby's heart rate, I would like to use fetal scalp blood sampling to determine fetal distress before doing a cesarean.

EPIDURALS

___ If an epidural is needed, I would like to request a low-dose epidural.

___ Please physically assist me to change positions with an epidural, including positions such as being on hands and knees, squatting, sitting fully upright, or sitting out of bed (and standing or walking if permitted by this facility).

___ If an epidural is used, please remember to continue providing massage and emotional support.

**CESAREANS**

___ During a cesarean, I would like to play music CDs (or a HypnoBirthing® CD) in the operating room.

___ Please describe the surgery and birth to me as it is happening.

___ Please do not describe the surgery in detail.

___ Please allow the baby to stay in the operating room until the surgery is over; please do not take the baby to the nursery if he or she is healthy.

___ If allowed, I would like my doula to be present for a cesarean. *(This is in addition to a family member, who will usually be permitted.)*

**THE UNEXPECTED**

___ I may need time to adjust if unexpected procedures are necessary. If it is not an emergency, please allow me to have (circle) 15/30/60 minutes before starting an unplanned procedure.

___ Please explain in detail why a procedure is needed and how it is performed so I can make a more informed decision.

___ It is helpful for me to talk about my emotions when I am stressed. Please ask me how I am feeling or coping if unexpected circumstances arise.

___ I may be anxious in the following situations and would like extra emotional support if they occur (circle): having an epidural/not having an epidural/having a cesarean/having a repeat cesarean/other: _____.

**CONTACT WITH BABY**

*In many hospitals, it is common for the staff to separate mothers and babies for bathing and routine exams shortly after birth. You may wish to request that these separations be minimized in any of the following ways.*

___ Please perform the first baby exam in my arms, not on a warming table.

___ Please encourage me to have skin contact with my baby and do not wrap my baby.

___ Please allow me to breastfeed my baby before she or he leaves my arms for the first time.

___ Please allow my baby to remain with me for at least (circle) one hour/two hours after birth, before taking my baby to the nursery.

___ I would like to come with my baby to the nursery for bathing or routine care right after birth, rather than being separated from my baby.

___ Please do not take my baby to the nursery for bathing or other nonemergency care right after birth.

**OTHER**

My other wishes for my birth are:

_____

_____

_____

_____

*From* **The Doula Guide to Birth** *by Lowe and Zimmerman. May be copied for individual use.*

## SAMPLE BIRTH PLANS

Following are two sample birth plans, in which we selected a few priorities that might be most important for these imaginary families.

### Sample Birth Plan #1

My name is Genevieve Henrard, and I will be supported in labor by my partner, Chris Green, and my doula, Gloria Jackson. I was born in France, where my mother gave birth to me with a *sage femme,* a person similar to a doula, and I am excited to be having this experience now. I would very much like to have natural childbirth (but if pain medicine is necessary, I would like the option of IV narcotics).

These other wishes are important to me:

1. I would like to request a room with a tub, if available when I arrive. Please encourage me to use the tub for pain relief often! Also, if labor seems slow, I would like to use the tub for ninety minutes, rather than using Pitocin right away.
2. A vaginal exam upon being admitted is fine. Please, no other vaginal exams unless medically urgent.
3. I have been practicing the squatting position and I would love to use it to push the baby out, or another upright position so I am not lying on my back.
4. In case of narcotics or an epidural, please help me with squatting, if I am able to, or lying on my side to push.
5. In case of cesarean, please allow my partner and my doula to both accompany me for emotional support, if possible. My doula has attended cesareans at this hospital and she is respectful of your operating room protocols.

I am thankful for all of your help!

## Sample Birth Plan #2

My name is Martha Cunningham, and I will be giving birth with my mother, Mary Cunningham, and my baby's father, Mark Jones. Mark and I both work as scientists at the university associated with this hospital, and this is our first baby. I have written the following birth plan and discussed it with my doctor in advance, and I appreciate your help with my wishes.

1. I expect that I'll use an epidural at some point. I'd like to delay it as long as I can, to minimize the amount of medication that might reach the baby.
2. I am open to a medical student being present; however, please explain to me clearly who each person in the room is.
3. Mark would like to help cut the baby's cord.
4. Please perform all routine baby exams with the baby in my arms in bed, not on a warming table.
5. In case of a cesarean, please allow the baby to stay in the operating room with me until the end of surgery. I understand that babies usually go to the nursery, but it's my hope that he can remain with me if he is healthy.

## PLANS FOR TWINS AND MULTIPLES

If you are expecting twins or multiples, your body is designed to go through labor with them in generally the same way as a singleton baby. However, many hospitals manage the births of multiples in a more highly medicalized way. It is important to know the protocols of your facility regarding multiples, as well as to think about your options and requests for labor, and to include these wishes in your written birth plan.

According to the American College of Obstetricians and Gynecologists (ACOG), 3 percent of all births consist of multiple babies. Most research that exists on women expecting multiples has looked at their pregnancies, not their births, and it has not been possible to base much of what is practiced in labor on scientific studies. Twins and multiples, along with their mothers, are somewhat more likely to experience health problems during pregnancy, birth, and postpartum, which has led to the increased medicalization of their care. For example, these families are more likely to experience prematurity, pregnancy-related hypertension, and babies admitted to the intensive care unit.

On the other hand, the majority of twin pregnancies are eligible for a normal vaginal birth, and numerous mothers have had natural childbirth with twins. The studies that do exist have not conclusively proven that a more medicalized approach results in healthier outcomes.

This section will mostly address women expecting twins, because the births of higher-order multiples are now routinely conducted by cesarean. However, in regard to higher-order multiples ACOG has stated: "there are retrospective case series that validate vaginal delivery as a potential mode of delivery, especially for triplet gestations." For mothers expecting triplets who are able to find practitioners who can deliver their babies vaginally, the information presented here may be adapted for them as well.

---

The following practices have been implemented by many hospitals and providers in regard to twin deliveries. According to ACOG and the Society of Obstetricians and Gynaecologists of Canada, most of these protocols are *not* supported by scientific research, but have nonetheless come to be accepted as the standard of care. These practices may include:

- Routinely inducing labor before thirty-seven weeks (This has been shown to increase breathing problems in newborn twins.)

- Routinely inducing labor at thirty-seven weeks (According to ACOG, pregnancy can continue for twins and mothers who are healthy at thirty-seven weeks.)
- Requiring an epidural (This is because without an epidural, the chance of needing general anesthesia with twins is slightly higher at 6 or 7 percent than with a singleton. But ultimately, the decision about an epidural belongs to the woman.)
- Requiring the mother to be constantly attached to a monitor for the babies' heartbeats, rather than listening at regular intervals (This protocol for twins was adopted in response to lawsuits, not medical research.)
- Routinely scheduling a cesarean even when the first baby is head down (Studies show scheduled cesareans do not offer increased benefits, regardless of whether the second baby is head down or breech.)
- For a vaginal delivery, having the mother push in the operating room rather than a normal labor room, because of a slightly increased need for cesarean sections.
- Routinely using interventions to speed up pushing of the second twin (Research shows this does not increase benefits to the baby except in cases of fetal distress.)

The above procedures may, of course, be medically necessary in individual cases. You have the right to decline their *routine* use after discussing the benefits, risks, and alternatives with your provider. We spoke with Kimberly Packard, a Massachusetts doula specializing in twin births, and also the mother of twins herself. Because hospital protocols for twins can be significantly more strict than for single babies, Kim advises mothers to choose their priorities and speak up for them, while recognizing that more compromises may be necessary.

When writing your wishes for a labor with twins, keep in mind some of the options from our standard birth plan checklist. For example, because of hospital practices that may increase the use of epidurals, Pitocin, and monitoring of the babies' heartbeats, you may especially want to consider asking for help with position changes, using a portable wireless monitor, and strategies to make these interventions a more positive experience.

There may also be additional doctors and nurses required at the birth of twins, which can add to a sense of commotion and noisiness. There can be a feeling of urgency or crisis in the room, even when the birth is proceeding normally. As part of your written birth plan, you may wish to ask that staff who are not essential in the moment remain quietly in the background.

You may be able to request that you stay in a regular labor room to give birth, rather than pushing in an operating room. Or, if you are required to push in the OR, you can request to remain on your delivery bed and not be transferred to an operating table for pushing, which is less comfortable. Operating rooms are usually brightly lit and stark in atmosphere. You can request that lights be kept dim during pushing and that music CDs be played.

Parents of twins may want to consider having two doulas. Because of the higher level of medicalization of these births, the additional emotional support may help diffuse some of the extra tension that can be present. While you are pregnant, you can also join Internet discussion groups with the National Organization of Mothers of Twins Clubs at www.nomotc.org, and hear stories from other women about how they negotiated their needs during labor. Congratulations on the birth of your babies!

## THE BIRTH ESSAY

The birth essay is another document you can write to communicate your needs with those who are caring for you in labor. It is used differently than a birth plan. A birth plan addresses practical issues, medical procedures, labor techniques, and your requests about *what will happen* during birth. A birth essay, on the other hand, is a tool to help you discover and share *how you feel* about your upcoming labor.

By writing about your emotions regarding birth, you may be able to reach an even deeper understanding of what you'll truly need as a laboring mother. And though many caregivers are surprisingly unfamiliar with techniques for emotionally supporting pregnant women, the birth essay can open lines of communication that allow providers to respond more deeply to their patients' needs, too.

Several practitioners have developed suggested guidelines for writing a birth essay, including Michele Helgeson, CNM, a midwife in the Boston area who has practiced in hospitals and an alternative birth center for over two decades. She describes her experience by saying: "The birth essay has, by far, proven to be the single most useful tool that I have in rendering emotional care to pregnant women."

To create your birth essay, allow yourself to write whatever comes to mind, for as long as you need, without worrying about spelling, grammar, or getting any answers "right." If you are familiar with the idea of a stream of consciousness, you can use your birth essay to express any and all thoughts that arise as you write. Some questions to help you get started are:

- What do you imagine it will be like going into labor, giving birth, and being with your new baby right after birth?
- What will giving birth mean to you, your baby, and your family?

- What are your dreams for your birth? What are your fears about giving birth?

We encourage you to write as *much* as possible in a birth essay, making it different from a birth plan, which is usually more useful if it is shorter. Writing a birth essay is like writing in a diary, a journal, a blog, or a letter to a good friend. If you don't have much experience with this type of writing, you can gently push yourself to keep going beyond the first page or two.

You may find that in writing a birth essay, you do wind up addressing some of the same issues as those that appear in a birth plan, such as your emotions about handling the pain of labor. It's fine if this happens. But you'll probably find yourself writing about a broader range of topics in a birth essay, including such things as feelings of happiness or sadness, your memories about the past, and your hopes for the future.

When you feel that you've finished writing, you have several choices about how to use your essay. You may feel comfortable sharing it with people such as your partner, a family member, a friend, or a counselor. Most doulas strive to be aware of the emotional needs of their clients, and would be interested in discussing your birth essay; this will also allow them to support you more knowledgeably during labor.

You may also wish to share your essay with your doctor or midwife. You do not have to actually give your "diary" to them, though you are welcome to show them what you wrote if you feel comfortable. Many providers are not familiar with the idea of a birth essay. However, it is fine to let your caregiver know that you have emotional concerns you would like to discuss, which may arise from writing your essay. You might want to read the essay aloud, or tell your provider what you wrote about, without presenting the actual pages to her.

By understanding your emotions, your providers have a better chance of fulfilling both your medical and personal wishes. Ask your provider for a longer appointment when you are ready to discuss your birth essay and your birth plan. Our hope is that these documents can be tools for your own self-discovery, and tools of discovery for your caregivers in their efforts to provide you and other women with the most compassionate care possible.

12

# Get Ready Now: What Really Happens Postpartum

There's a moment, shortly after giving birth, that many new mothers remember vividly. It comes after the thrill of the birth event begins to subside, and as you start taking stock of your post-marathon body and new-mom brain. It comes after you've marveled over your swaddled child asleep in her little bassinet. Suddenly, you are jolted by a simple thought: there is now a tiny, helpless creature dependent on your unconditional love for survival. You have to function as a responsible adult; there's no going back.

Before she was born, you may have done yoga, taken extra

folic acid, and laid the mental and physical foundation for labor and birth. But in your excitement, you understandably may not have spent much time thinking about the workload of postpartum life: according to La Leche League, feeding a newborn takes forty hours a week or more. You'll change multiple diapers a day, wash several loads of laundry, and you will handle these new responsibilities in a sleep-deprived state.

## ⚮ ADOPTION ⚮

If you are a mother placing your baby for adoption or you are a surrogate mother, you may be interested in reading these pages to learn what life will be like for your baby during the early weeks of life with his new family. Also, please see the section titled "Doula Specialty: Adoption and Surrogacy" in chapter 5 for information about how your doula can be helpful to you postpartum, and for other resources for birth mothers.

When this reality begins to sink in, you may be surprised to discover darker thoughts and feelings lurking around: exhaustion, a sense of being overwhelmed, and, as the newborn's primary caregiver, isolation.

If you harbored a fantasy of your new family cocooned in a clean house and eating healthy delicious food together, the postpartum reality may feel unmanageable and disappointing. Of course, for most of us, there will be surges of elation and love for the child. But many new moms also quietly wonder, "Why isn't this easier? Why is mothering not coming naturally? Why are my partner and I not on the same wavelength?"

You may feel like Helene, the chief financial officer of a small publishing company in New York, who now has two young children. "I am a high-functioning, very competent businessperson who was totally and completely overwhelmed by dealing with an infant," she says. "There is a culture of competence that makes it somehow unacceptable to discuss how difficult everything is among peers."

## WHAT YOUR BIRTH DOULA CAN DO POSTPARTUM

Doulas are aware that the postpartum season sometimes is a tough one. However, with a bit of pre-birth planning and a frank assessment of what your new (and substantial) needs will be, your doula can help you cope with the postpartum period and enjoy its tenderness.

Just as your birth plan helped define your desires about birth, a *postpartum plan* crafted with the help of your doula can make this time more manageable. Focusing on your postpartum life well before it arrives is key. The things that help most are fairly low tech and designed to get your basic needs met: sleeping, eating, connecting with your baby, and making sure that your emotional support system is strong. All of this should soften your landing into new motherhood.

We think of the postpartum period as the time from birth until the baby gets into a regular sleep routine (with "regular" and "routine" broadly defined). Usually it takes at least three to five months (but sometimes longer) to establish a pattern of sorts with extended periods of sleep at night and shorter naps during the day. When you get that first long nighttime sleep (five to six hours), it feels like a miracle (that is, after you reassure yourself that the baby hasn't stopped breathing).

Most birth doulas will visit you postpartum—shortly after the birth, perhaps while you're still in the hospital, or at home. The home visit is designed to make sure your plan is working and to answer—or find the person who can answer—

any questions you might have. Doulas also review the birth, find out how your mood is, and provide referrals to counselors and support groups for depression or help with breastfeeding. (It's worth asking in advance if your doula is a lactation consultant—many are.)

Eliza, a nutritionist and mother of two says, "I found I really needed to go over every intimate detail of the birth with my doula a few times since I was so floored by it all." Some doulas try to take notes during birth in order to help you process the experience later.

Leah Kohlstrom, a doula in Camden, Maine, says expectant moms (especially first-timers) are sometimes so focused on the birth that they can't think beyond that point. Many are simply too overloaded to plan in the same way for the postpartum period. Still, at thirty-five or thirty-six weeks, she advises pregnant women and their partners to devise a simple postpartum plan to cover the basics.

The benefits of planning are worthwhile. Megan and Rose, the couple from chapter 2, describe their experience:

> Postpartum was easier than we expected, even with twins. While Megan was pregnant, our birth doula helped us figure out that we could find a part-time family helper to live in our spare room, in exchange for room and board rather than pay. This was a really affordable way for us to get the support we needed, and it made all the difference.

## SLEEP

When you're in college, pulling an all-nighter to cram for a midterm, or salsa dancing until four AM is no big deal. It's actually kind of a thrill. But after birth, when your body is sore, and there's a baby sucking on you every two hours, twenty-four hours a day, and no one really "gets" what you're going through, loss of sleep can push you over an emotional cliff. And while new mothers, of course, are most affected by postpartum sleep deprivation, fathers and partners are not immune, particularly those who return to work quickly and lose the opportunity for daytime naps. "I never even realized I could be so exhausted," said a thirty-eight-year-old father, an engineer, who had spent his earlier years in graduate school functioning at a high level on four hours of sleep per night.

Sleep disruption in general has been linked to a range of physical and mental illness, including diabetes, obesity, and depression. It has also been associated with deficits of short-term memory, reaction time, and motor skills—all critical for taking care of a new baby.

From our perspective, getting enough sleep is the most important tool you've got for managing the postpartum period. Without it, those weeks can feel unendurable and getting back to "normal life" nearly impossible. But if you figure out a way to protect your sleep, you can begin to savor new motherhood, bond with your baby, and reestablish your relationship with your partner and your work.

Of course, everyone says you should sleep when your baby sleeps. But that isn't so easy because we live in a culture where there is always something "more important" to do. Actually, there isn't! Your doula will encourage you to think through exactly what might stop you from lying down when your baby does.

If it's cleaning the house, you can either figure out a way for someone else to take over some of the cleaning, or you might relax your standards. If it's doing the dishes, your doula might encourage you to use disposable plates, napkins, and utensils. "A lot of women in Maine use cloth diapers," says Ms. Kohlstrom, the Camden doula. But she encourages them to go for disposables—at least temporarily until their domestic life is a bit calmer. Alternatively, hire a diaper service or request it as a gift.

Experienced doulas can help you begin to establish a

nighttime sleep routine—for the baby as well as the rest of the family. This is not a simple process. Half a dozen books try to teach you how, but from our perspective, having an expert problem-solve with you in real time is more effective.

Don't fixate on an idealized notion of how your family will sleep. We don't know many families that sleep in that iconic way families are supposed to: with the newborn in a cradle in the bedroom, older child soundly snoozing in her room, and Mom and Dad snuggling in bed. Women and couples must figure out what allows them to get the most sleep possible and sometimes it's not obvious or conventional.

Jennifer Fargár, an Atlanta doula with a young son, says she didn't realize she was a "princess, who needs eight hours of sleep and total darkness," until she had a baby and lost her delicious, uninterrupted sleep. In order to function as a mother and caregiver she ended up sharing a bed with her baby so she could nurse him through the night without getting up. But for her husband, a light sleeper, that plan was untenable. He slept upstairs for six months. "I was kind of disappointed," she said. "But that's what worked for us." Learn to be flexible; let go of your original plan if it is causing stress.

Some couples solve the sleep problem by sharing the work. One couple split the nights in half: Mom nursed the baby at ten PM and then slept until four AM. Dad handled the midnight and two AM feedings using pumped milk and handed the baby back to Mom at four AM so he could sleep until ten AM. Another couple alternated entire nights so each one got at least six hours every other night.

Even if you don't delegate night feedings, decide in advance who will get up with the baby in the night if she wakes up, and who gets up first in the morning. "I found it easier to roll over and sleep through baby cries when I knew I was off the hook," says one mother. Having a plan can also prevent cranky, middle-of-the-night arguments with your partner.

Single parents will likely have to do even more preparing.

During her son's first few weeks of life, Janet, a single mother, turned for guidance to her birth doula, who is also a lactation consultant:

> My doula said I could call her every day if I had questions. Sleeping was hard at first, and she suggested I wake the baby during the day and give him a couple of extra feedings. When I did that, the baby needed fewer feedings in the middle of the night. That really helped, and I never would have realized you could do that, if she hadn't been there for me to call.

If you are serious about sleep and can budget for it, night nurses, overnight nannies, and nighttime postpartum doulas are available to lovingly handle your baby through much of the night. They also help teach you about healthy sleep routines, scheduling options, swaddling, and other skills. Consider hiring a service for even one night a week through several weeks or asking a friend or relative to do an overnight.

Sharon Davis, a doula in Holland, Massachusetts, describes how she works with mothers to help devise a sleep plan that also promotes breastfeeding. For one family, Ms. Davis stayed with the new baby in a separate room until it was time for him to breastfeed, trying to give the mother as much time as possible between feedings by rocking and cuddling the infant. When it was time, Ms. Davis would change the baby and then bring him to the mother, who was sleeping in the bedroom. Ms. Davis would leave, close the door, and return to the guest room. When the feeding was over, she'd collect the infant and bring him back to the other room to sleep—usually on her own chest!

Kathleen Sullivan, a postpartum doula in Los Angeles works with families for the first three months after birth. She says she tries to help parents establish daily routines for sleeping, eating, and bathing so that babies begin to know what to expect. "It's all about looking at a newborn from their perspective," she says, explaining her motto: "Schedules are for parents, routines are for babies."

If you are able to hire a nighttime support person, do not feel guilty. It is temporary and you are preserving your body and your sanity in order to be a better provider for your baby.

And what works for one baby may not for another. Miranda, a librarian, hired a postpartum doula to work nights when her first son was born. The doula came several nights a week, from eleven PM until seven AM and fed the baby a bottle of either pumped milk or formula while she and her husband slept. "I would usually get up once in the middle of the night to pump," Miranda said. "Still, it felt luxurious." When she was pregnant with her second child, the couple once again hired a postpartum doula, expecting the same schedule. But their second son, while a much better sleeper than his older brother, refused to take a bottle, despite myriad feeding strategies and experiments with different nipples. "I really couldn't go anywhere or do anything," Miranda said. Eventually, they had to change their approach and the doula's responsibilities. "She would come over during the day and keep the baby reasonably content so I could take a walk," Miranda said. "In a way it was frustrating, and also funny; we thought we already knew what the issues were."

One mother of twins said the best sleep advice she got was to stay in bed until she amassed the correct amount of hours, even if it took twelve hours to sleep six or eight. "Leave blinds drawn, stay in PJs and do infant care, then sleep, then infant care, then sleep until you have cobbled enough together."

## SLEEP, DEPRESSION,
### AND WELL-BEING

Up to 85 percent of all new mothers in the U.S. experience postpartum "blues" during the first ten days or so after birth. And at some point during the first twelve months, between 10 and 20 percent of new mothers, as many as 850,000 women in the U.S., experience diagnosable postpartum depression. We're not saying that sleep alone can cure true depression in new mothers, but it can certainly help.

According to research explored in the book *Sleep Disorders in Women: A Guide to Practical Management (Current Clinical Neurology)*, "Increased sleep, which can be improved with daytime activities such as light exposure and exercise, may be more therapeutic in treating the depressed state than counseling, psychotherapy or antidepressant medication." Researchers also found that being in labor during the night, coupled with sleep disruption at the end of pregnancy, might result in a higher incidence of postpartum blues.

In a large survey in 2007 called "Sleep in America," the National Sleep Foundation concluded what most new mothers know all too well: "Poor sleep is associated with poor mood." Among postpartum women in the study, 42 percent report that they rarely or never get a good night's sleep—the highest frequency of all the groups of women surveyed. When asked what awakens them most during the night, 90 percent of postpartum women say giving care to a child. Nearly one-half of postpartum women say that they have no one helping them with child care at night.

Sleep also helps strengthen your emerging role as a primary caretaker.

A study published in 2007 in the *Journal of Perinatal & Neonatal Nursing* discusses the steps involved in one of the most profound transformations in life: becoming a mother. It describes four overlapping stages in the process: "committing, attaching and preparing for the infant during pregnancy; becoming acquainted and attached with the infant, including learning how to care for the infant and restoring maternal health; moving toward a 'new normal'; and achieving a maternal identity."

The nurse and midwife team who conducted the qualitative study write that developing a "sleep-consciousness"—which basically means learning how to get adequate sleep and knowing what can happen if you don't—plays a major role in whether new mothers are able to integrate these stages and restore their mental and physical health.

## FOOD

Without food, moms get cranky and tired, and sometimes so frustrated that they can't nurse. Don't fall into this cycle. You need protein, carbohydrates, fresh fruits, vegetables, and calcium in the form of tasty, healthful snacks. And despite the reality that you are probably carrying around a good deal of extra weight, this is not the time to diet. You need energy!

A few weeks before you have the baby, prepare some simple dishes that can be doubled—lasagna, burritos, soups, potpies—

and freeze the extra portions. Stock up on simple, nutritious foods: yogurt, baby carrots, fruits, nuts, hard-boiled eggs—that can give you a quick fix and that you can eat easily before climbing back into bed. (See section on sleep, above.)

Ask friends and relatives eager to help out to prepare a meal or two. This will make all of you happy. Consider a local organic produce delivery service and stock up on take-out menus. If you feel you are too tired or distracted to eat, ask your partner or close friend to make it their focus to keep you fed.

## CHORES

When a friend, relative, or neighbor calls and says, "What can I do?" *never* say nothing. Jennifer Fargár, the Atlanta doula, encourages her clients to make a list of every task involved in running the house, from bringing in the mail or dumping the bathroom garbage to laundry, dishes, picking up or dropping off an older child at school, or walking the dog. Arrange your house so it's easy for someone else to handle these tasks and remember, they're eager to help! "People want to do more than just bring over a cute baby outfit," Ms. Fargar says.

Decide in advance who is planning to come "visit" and who is planning to come "help." The visitors can wait a few weeks until you've gotten to know your new baby and are feeling stronger. Trisha, who worked as the manager of a farm stand until the birth of her son, now five months old, said her mother came for three weeks and "did everything—cooked, cleaned, did the laundry, shopped, and rented a car, which we don't have. It was unbelievable. I'd wake up and breakfast would be made."

If you don't think your own mother will be quite so helpful, reassess your post-birth invitation list.

Think about whether your mother-in-law will really help take care of you. Do you feel comfortable asking her to do the laundry and vacuum? Will it be possible to leave her for long stretches while you and the baby rest? Remember, you are not a hostess right now.

## STAY CONNECTED

Whether you are taking a six-week maternity leave or becoming a stay-at-home mom, you will inevitably end up spending some long stretches alone with your newborn. This time together is precious—there is nothing more fascinating than getting to know your child, and snuggling alone with her is tremendously satisfying.

However, a few long days caring for an infant on your own can be grueling. And with little or no adult contact during the day, many new moms feel deeply isolated, or even slip into depression.

Doulas are like the postpartum Welcome Wagon, showing up at your door with resources to help you connect with the new community you now find yourself in. Get involved by reaching out to other new mothers and identifying support services before your baby is born. Stay in touch with people at work, even if you're taking an extended leave. Plan dates and reconnect with friends. If your birth was traumatic, find a professional to talk through it in detail with you.

By attending even one meeting of the breastfeeding support group La Leche League while you're pregnant, you give yourself a lifeline if things look bleak postpartum. You know there is always someone you can call. The Web site of the magazine for natural family living, www.mothering.com, has "tribes" and regional resources. Or just visit www.craigslist .org, the Web site with classified ads for cities around the world, to find playdates or other moms nearby who want to join you in a local park. Some independent toy stores have new moms groups and many public libraries host sing-alongs for all ages. In many cities, organizations such as Jewish Family

Service offer new mom discussion groups, and will connect you to experts who can help with sleep, breastfeeding, and other issues.

When you're ready, getting exercise alone or in a group can preserve your sanity. Some gyms offer on-site babysitting. Even one hour a day outside your house with other moms can completely restore your perspective.

Some groups have a special focus, such as teaching infant massage or addressing depression. Patricia Arcari, a nurse-scientist, leads a program called Calm Mother, Happy Child at the Benson-Henry Institute for Mind Body Medicine at Massachusetts General Hospital in Boston. The class begins each week with relaxation exercises and meditation. The group focuses on what Ms. Arcari calls "mindful mothering," which attempts to help women feel more grounded and deepen the joy and satisfaction of mothering in all stages. Caretaking is stressful, and frequently, physical symptoms flare, including sleep problems, headaches, and anxiety. Ms. Arcari's class focuses on how to alleviate these physical symptoms through relaxation, breathing, meditation, physical exercise, and nutrition in a climate of social supportiveness and sharing.

## YOUR RELATIONSHIP

A number of books in the past few years have brought into focus a dilemma for those who are married or partnered: how to keep your relationship intact after the birth of a baby. *Babyproofing Your Marriage, And Baby Makes Three,* and *Mating in Captivity* are just a few of the titles that suggest couples are growing more aware and open about the challenges in their relationships after children.

A study published in 2000 in the *Journal of Family Psychology* found that two-thirds of couples experience a significant decline in marriage satisfaction—including less-frequent or less-satisfying sex, more conflict, and more emotional distance—after the first baby arrives. The study, funded by the National

Institute of Mental Health, involved tracking eighty-two new-lywed couples (forty-nine of which became pregnant) for four to six years. This research confirmed earlier findings about marital happiness after children are born.

Becoming a parent is life-altering: your priorities and interests shift, sometimes so dramatically that it seems you've developed a new personality. A job that may have defined you suddenly becomes less important. The adrenaline rush you craved while working against deadlines or making deals may no longer be attractive. Exotic travel, once alluring, may now feel like a drag.

Sometimes, the person whom you had a child with may also seem less attractive. A new mother recalls her disappointment that the man she thought would be her true partner as a parent didn't take on his share of chores, and seemed uninterested in many of the details of newborn life. This led her to withdraw, and their intimacy dwindled.

Research—and plain common sense—suggests that when a couple's sex life diminishes, their deepest bonds can also start to unravel. While some women want to get back to sexual activity shortly after birth, many say it's the last thing they want after all of the other demands on their body. Some couples start slowly, initiating other types of intimate activity, like kissing and cuddling, but not having sex. The main point here is that while some couples will be on the same wavelength sexually at this time, far more won't be: most studies suggest men want sex—and more of it—shortly after birth while women need more time. Still, this topic will require some discussion and probably some work after the baby is born, so don't ignore it.

Couples therapy before the baby is born and early postpartum is a good place to get support. If therapy isn't feasible, remember to try to set aside time to talk to each other, offer praise for the hard work you are both doing, and give each other the benefit of the doubt.

When your body has recovered, sex—even quick, less-than-fabulous sex—can help give both of you a visceral memory of the romance of life before kids. When you're ready, start thinking about regular date nights.

Of course, restoring your relationship isn't all about sex. It's also about keeping in mind why you are a couple in the first place, what your common interests and passions are, and continuing to enjoy them.

## CALL IN THE EXPERTS

If harmonizing your sleep, meals, chores, and key relationships still seems too overwhelming, look into hiring a postpartum doula. Some European countries automatically provide this kind of professional support for new families, while U.S. mothers have to seek it out.

A little bit Mary Poppins, a little bit loving Mom, an experienced postpartum doula can truly help you feel like you are getting your life back.

Indeed, postpartum doulas have a broad job description: their basic responsibilities can involve breastfeeding/baby-feeding support, baby care while the mother rests or showers, laundry, trash removal, teaching parents how to swaddle or soothe the baby, older sibling care, grocery shopping, and pet care. But their reach can go much further: they can help you find natural remedies for healing hemorrhoids, or wait in the car with your newborn when you take that first post-birth yoga class. They can make you a tofu stir-fry and your husband a beef lasagna. They can steer you to marriage counselors and sleep consultants.

Postpartum doulas charge around $25 to $40 an hour in big U.S. cities. Rates tend to be higher for twins or multiples and some doulas specialize in multiple babies. Prices can also depend on the range of duties: for instance, whether the postpartum doula is doing a lot of cooking. A limited number of hospitals, birth centers, and community programs make postpartum doulas available at no charge, particularly to low-income families.

You can find a postpartum doula through word of mouth, the Internet, or go through an agency, such as MotherCare Services, Inc., which operates in the greater Boston area, and was founded in the mid-1980s by Joan Singer, one of the pioneers in the postpartum doula movement. Ms. Singer does an initial needs assessment and matches mothers with doulas who can best fulfill those needs.

Finding a postpartum doula who can alleviate the stress of new motherhood by allowing you to focus on nurturing the baby and recuperating physically can stave off depression and allow intimate bonding to begin.

Women rank postpartum doula services as one of the best gifts they've ever received. A mother of three raves that her postpartum doula turned out to be of more assistance than her mother: "She was there just to help me, and that, quite simply, saved my life."

Belinda, a first-time mom, tells her story:

> My in-laws came to stay and meet the baby about a week in. They helped care for her, and my husband helped care for them . . . but no one was really looking after me. At about three weeks my in-laws left and my husband went back to work. I was afraid to take care of the baby all by myself. I was recovering from a difficult pregnancy and had torn during labor, and I really needed some nurturing as well. Our doula was a gift from my mother, hired ostensibly to care for the baby but she did wonderful little things for me as well, like bringing me water and snacks when I sat down to nurse, and teaching me how to use my breast pump and swaddle the baby. The main thing was that she was so calm and collected and I was so nervous. I was struggling to

breastfeed and I didn't know how to hold my daughter properly and my breasts were humongous. I was physically and emotionally so vulnerable, and she was so respectful of what I was going through.

## WHEN THE UNEXPECTED HAPPENS

There are many reasons that your plans for a smooth postpartum period might get upended. And as a mother of two says: "It's never the thing you think will go wrong that does."

One in three women in the U.S. now gives birth by cesarean section, major surgery that significantly lengthens postpartum recovery time. These mothers won't be able to drive for about a month and lifting will be difficult for some time. In this situation it is even more important to have backup help. Doulas will give you ideas on how to get this support, for instance a father might be eligible for a longer family medical leave from work if the mother underwent surgery.

If the new parents didn't plan on having visitors or postpartum help, we recommend they do have a plan B in case of emergency. Perhaps they want to designate a close friend or relative as the visitor/helper only if an emergency arises. For instance, if the mother or baby must return for many doctor's appointments after discharge, or if one of them is rehospitalized, then extra postpartum help will be needed.

Even without a medical emergency, you may find you need extra help. Greta, a therapist who had done extensive research on birth and parenting before she had her first child at home at age thirty-nine, never imagined breastfeeding would be a problem. But on her son's second day of life, he began crying—and didn't stop for about twelve hours. "We had no idea what was wrong with him," she recalls. She noticed the business card of a lactation consultant lying around her house, and in her fraught state, picked up the phone. The consultant came over, and helped Greta feed the baby breast milk through a straw and then taught him how to latch on properly. The household suddenly got calm. "Here I am with a PhD and nearly forty years of life experience and I couldn't tell my baby was hungry," Greta says. "The lactation consultant saved us." When she had her second child, breastfeeding came naturally, and Greta happily nursed her daughter until her third birthday.

## LIFE GOES ON

The postpartum period will soon slip into a new phase where you are more confident and settled as a mother and in tune with your baby. Congratulations! You are now well into parenthood, the most amazing, complex, humbling, and gratifying job you'll ever have. If the stories in these pages have a moral, it would be to try to learn and plan as much as you can before your child is born, and then let it all go and be open to the daily joys, frustrations, and completely unexpected twists her arrival will bring. When you're not sure where to turn postpartum, check in with your birth doula for ideas, even if months have passed since your baby was born. Remember to keep some perspective, find humor in the middle of the night, and cherish your newborn because she's probably the closest you will ever come to pure magic in your short time here on earth.

# APPENDIX

## EVALUATION OF YOUR BIRTH

*From* The Doula Guide to Birth *by Lowe and Zimmerman.*
*May be copied for individual use.*

You may fill out this form and share it with your provider, your doula, or a counselor as a way to discuss your feelings after your birth and your current needs regarding it.

Your name: _____
Baby's name: _____

### Hopes and Expectations

(For each of the following questions, please choose from these answers: far less than I expected/somewhat less/about as much as I expected/somewhat more/far more.)

- The length of labor was:
- The pain or sensation of labor was:
- The amount of pain drugs used in labor was:
- The amount of other medical interventions used in labor was:

- The amount of time my caregivers spent with me in labor was:
- Breastfeeding has worked out:

1. I felt my caregivers listened to my expectations for birth and tried to fulfill them. (yes/no)
2. If my expectations could not be met, I felt included in decisions about my care. (yes/no)
3. I felt informed about why any medical procedures were needed. (yes/no)
4. My caregivers obtained my agreement before performing any medical procedures. (yes/no)
5. I feel that medical procedures I received were necessary. (yes/no/unsure)
6. If I planned a VBAC, I birthed vaginally. (yes/no)
7. I received enough encouragement and support to help me cope with the pain of labor. (yes/no)
8. I received enough encouragement and support to help me succeed with breastfeeding. (yes/no)

### The Unexpected

Unexpected events that happened during my birth included (circle any that apply):

baby needing intensive care or special care

cesarean

death of baby

epidural

epidural not working

episiotomy

fetal distress

fever in labor

forceps

general anesthesia

induction

narcotics

not getting an epidural that I wanted

Pitocin

premature baby

unexpected breech

unexpected disability or illness in baby

vacuum

other:_____

I experienced events that increased the normal pain of labor (circle any that apply):

| | |
|---|---|
| back labor | not being allowed to leave my |
| being sleep-deprived | bed |
| extreme hunger | Pitocin |
| extreme nausea | other: _____ |

I felt prepared in advance for unplanned events in labor. (yes/no)

### Emotions I Experienced

At some point during my birth I felt (circle any that apply):

| | |
|---|---|
| calm | loved |
| capable | nervous |
| challenged by the pain | respected |
| discouraged | sad |
| disrespected | tense |
| excited | terrified |
| extreme suffering | thrilled |
| happy | worried about my baby |
| helpless | other: _____ |
| in control | |

If I had an epidural, when the decision was made I felt (circle any that apply):

| | |
|---|---|
| accepting | pressure not to have it |
| afraid | pressure to have it |
| angry | relieved |
| disappointed | supported |
| failure or guilt | uncertain |

If I had a cesarean, when the decision was made I felt (circle any that apply):

| | |
|---|---|
| accepting | pressure not to have it |
| afraid | pressure to have it |
| angry | relieved |
| disappointed | supported |
| failure or guilt | uncertain |

I am proud of my body for (circle any that apply):
- growing my baby or multiples inside me
- starting labor on my own
- breaking my water on my own
- doing natural childbirth
- going through a short amount of labor
- going through a long amount of labor
- going through labor with Pitocin
- going through surgery
- pushing
- providing milk for my baby
- other:

I have experienced these possible signs of grief or trauma about my birth (circle any that apply):
- anger or irritability
- anxiety
- avoiding things that remind me of the birth, such as going near the hospital
- difficulty concentrating or making decisions
- feeling detached from my baby or loved ones
- feeling alone in my emotions
- insomnia or sleeping too much
- missing my baby (if separated from baby)
- poor appetite
- sadness

- urgently replaying the birth in my mind
- urgently trying to figure out "what went wrong" during birth

My current feelings about my birth can be described as:

great happiness                    great unhappiness
satisfaction                       I have mixed feelings
acceptance                         other: _____
dissatisfaction

# ENDNOTES

## Chapter 1

Page 10: A 2003 evaluation of the first four years of the community-based doula pilot project in Chicago . . .

Altfeld, S. *The Chicago Doula Project Evaluation Final Report.* The Ounce of Prevention Fund, 2003.

## Chapter 2

Page 28: A 2007 analysis funded by the National Institutes of Health . . .

Bronte-Tinkew, Jacinta, et al. 2007. "Men's Pregnancy Intentions and Prenatal Behaviors: What They Mean for Fathers' Involvement with Their Children." *Child Trends Research Brief.*

Page 28: Studies show fathers participate *more* when a doula is present.

Klaus, Marshall, et al. 1993. *Mothering the Mother,* p. 72. Reading, Massachusetts: Perseus Books.

Page 30: Over the years, books for gay families have occasionally appeared . . . Brill, Stephanie. 2006. *The New Essential*

*Guide to Lesbian Conception, Pregnancy & Birth.* New York: Alyson Books.

Page 31: Kitzinger, Sheila. 1996. *Becoming a Grandmother,* pp.15–16. New York: Fireside.

Page 36: A study of fourteen first-time fathers . . .

Chandler, Susan, et al. 1997. "Becoming a Father: First-time Fathers' Experience of Labor and Delivery." *Journal of Nurse-Midwifery,* vol. 42, issue one, pp.17–24; January.

## Chapter 3

Page 42: . . . Dr. Lamaze wrote that among the thousands of pregnant women he trained . . .

Lamaze, Fernand. 1984. *Painless Childbirth: The Lamaze Method.* Chicago: Contemporary Books.

Page 44: . . . Laura Shanley's Web site with a wealth of stories about sexuality in labor.

This Web site is dedicated to the option of giving birth at home "unassisted," that is, with no health-care provider present. Please note that we are not recommending giving birth at home with a doula as your *only* caregiver.

Page 53: *Thus, from 1951 to 1970, I saw hundreds of babies born.*

Sutton, Jean. 2003. "Birth Without Active Pushing." *Midwifery: Best Practice,* vol. 1: 90. Wickham, Sara, ed. Books For Midwives.

Page 55: When women were allowed to push without straining, the research showed "better progress and greater ease [that] has to be witnessed to be believed," and . . .

Beynon, Constance. 1957. "The Normal Second Stage of Labor: A Plea for Reform in Its Conduct." *Journal of Obstetrics and Gynaecology of the British Empire,* 64(6): 815–20.

## Chapter 4

Page 64: We spoke with anesthesiologist Dr. William Camann . . .

Camann, William, and Kathryn Alexander. 2006. *Easy Labor: Every Woman's Guide to Choosing Less Pain and More Joy During Childbirth.* New York: Ballantine Books.

## Chapter 5

Page 102: The editor of *Mothering* magazine called it "the best birth film ever made."

www.mothering.com/rickilakeinterview/

## Chapter 7

Page 120: Abnormal Symptoms in Early Labor

The information in this section is drawn from the following sources:

American College of Obstetricians and Gynecologists. 2007. *You and Your Baby: Prenatal Care, Labor and Delivery, and Postpartum Care,* Patient Education Pamphlet.

Cambridge Health Alliance Maternity Unit, Cambridge, MA. 2008. Discharge Instructions.

Janssen, Patricia, et al. 2007. "Early Labor Assessment and Support at Home Versus Telephone Triage: A Randomized Controlled Trial." *Obstetrical & Gynecological Survey,* 62(5), pp.287–288.

Mount Auburn Hospital, The Birth Place, Cambridge, MA. 2008. Discharge Instructions.

## Chapter 8

Page 125: *When I arrived at the hospital in labor with my doula, the doctor said my cervix was dilated about 6 centimeters. And it stayed that way for another twenty-four hours.*

This situation happened safely with natural childbirth, not Pitocin. Increasing levels of Pitocin with no dilation would not necessarily be safe for this long.

Page 131: **When time breaches in normal labor boundaries are the only pregnancy complications, interventions other than cesarean delivery must be considered before resorting to this method of delivery for failure to progress.**

Leveno, Kenneth, et al. 2003. *Williams Manual of Obstetrics,* twenty-first edition, p. 166. New York: McGraw-Hill.

Page 133: They concluded: "The increased risk of cesarean delivery was attributable to procedures performed for poor progress in labor."

Smith, Gordon, et al. 2008. "Cervical Length at Mid-Pregnancy and the Risk of Primary Cesarean Delivery." *New England Journal of Medicine,* 358:1346–53.

Page 137: *In the usual context of modern birth, it is the midwife's or the doctor's finger that gives information about the progress of labor.*

Odent, Michel. 2003. *Birth and Breastfeeding,* p. 42. East Sussex: Clairview Books.

Page 140: According to anthropologist Sheila Kitzinger, Jamaican midwives say, "The baby will not be born until the mother opens her back."

Sutton, Jean. 2003. "Birth Without Active Pushing." *Midwifery: Best Practice,* vol. 1: 90. Wickham, Sara, ed. Books For Midwives.

Page 140: She explains, "Your vagina is a lot like your nose— other people may do harm if they put fingers or instruments up there, but you have a greater sensitivity and will not do yourself any harm."

Lemay, Gloria. In the Midwife Archives Web site. 2008. www.gentlebirth.org/archives/birth.html#Self-Checking. Personal communication, May 19, 2008.

Page 141: However, more current research shows *the use of vaginal exams* is the primary factor that raises the risk of infection; the passing of time has not been shown to be the cause by itself.

Schutte, M., et al. 1983. "Management of Premature Rupture of Membranes: The Risk of Vaginal Examination to the Infant." *American Journal of Obstetrics & Gynecology,* 146(4): 395–400.

Page 143: However, *even the presence of GBS is a much lower risk factor* than having multiple vaginal exams in labor!

Seaward, P. Gareth, et al. 1997. "International Multicentre Term Prelabor Rupture of Membranes Study: Evaluation of predictors of clinical chorioamnionitis and postpartum fever in patients with prelabor rupture of membranes at term." *American Journal of Obstetrics & Gynecology,* 177(5): 1024–1029.

Page 147: "Repeated vaginal examinations are an invasive intervention of as yet no proved value. Those who advocate its use have the responsibility to test their belief in an appropriately controlled trial."

Enkin, Murray. 1992. "Commentary: 'Do I Do That? Do I Really Do That? Like That?'" *Birth,* 19(1): 19–21.

Page 150: According to the Cochrane Collaboration, studies involving over 58,000 women show that "the increase in cesarean section rate is much greater when scalp pH estimates are not available."

Enkin, Murray, et al. 2000. *A Guide to Effective Care in Pregnancy and Childbirth.* Third edition, p. 271. Oxford: Oxford University Press.

## Chapter 9

Page 160: . . . tools that may be available to assist you in positioning yourself include . . .

Rogers, Judith. 2005. *The Disabled Woman's Guide to Pregnancy and Birth*. New York: Demos Medical Publishing.

Page 160: *It is not merely a matter of "positions" for delivery, but of providing physical support for movement during contractions.*

Kitzinger, Sheila. 1997. "Authoritative Touch in Childbirth: A Cross-Cultural Approach." *Childbirth and Authoritative Knowledge*. Robbie Davis-Floyd and Carolyn Sargent, eds., p. 221. Berkeley, CA: University of California Press.

Page 173: *Some women stop eating or sleeping because they are excited and believe themselves to be in labor.*

Peterson, Gayle. 1993. *An Easier Childbirth*. Pp. 79–80. Berkeley, CA: Shadow and Light Publications.

Page 174: Besides helping you feel drowsy, alcohol is considered a *tocolytic,* or labor inhibitor, and may give you a couple of hours without contractions. (Historically, doctors gave it to mothers by IV to stop premature labors.)

Katz, Michael, et al., eds. 1988. *Preventing Preterm Birth: A Parent's Guide*. P. 95. San Francisco: Health Publishing Company.

## Chapter 10

Page 177: *The most important thing I learned when I was working as a nurse-midwife at an obstetric ward was that every mother wants to have a special, wonderful childbirth experience.*

Kishi, Rieko. 2005. "Supporting the Mother's Childbirth Experience." www.childresearch.net.

Page 179: Based on these findings, scientists from Belgium concluded in 2007, "the empowerment of laboring women, not the management of childbirth by means of painkillers, leads to satisfactory birth experiences."

Christiaens, Wendy, and Piet Bracke. 2007. "Assessment

of Social Psychological Determinants of Satisfaction with Childbirth in a Cross-National Perspective." *BMC Pregnancy and Childbirth,* 7: 26.

Page 179: "The decision to perform a cesarean section is one which the physician can make. The decision to have a cesarean birth is one which the parents should make."

Enkin, Murray. 1977. "Having a Section Is Having a Baby." *Birth and the Family Journal,* 4:2.

Page 180: *Childbirth is an experience of unrivaled vulnerability, encompassing all that is most personal and most precious . . .*

Radosti, Sue. 1999. "The Dynamics of Trauma in Childbirth." *Special Delivery,* vol. 22, no. 1, pp. 2–3.

Page 182: *Acknowledging fear can deepen our reserves and help us discover fresh meaning and commitment in our lives.*

Peterson, Gayle. 1993. *An Easier Childbirth.* Pp. 63–64. Berkeley, CA: Shadow and Light Publications.

### Chapter 11

Page 198: For examples of checklists that address topics beyond the scope of our book . . .

Wagner, Marsden. 2006. *Creating Your Birth Plan: The Definitive Guide to a Safe and Empowering Birth.* New York: Penguin Group.

Page 200: *With the exception of epidural use, doctors tend to manage labor the same way regardless of patient preferences.*

Greenfield, Marjorie. 2008. "Do Birth Plans Affect the Course of Labor?" http://health.yahoo.com/experts/pregnancy/3302/do-birth-plans-affect-the-course-of-labor.

Page 212: However, in regard to higher-order multiples ACOG has stated: "there are retrospective case series that validate vaginal delivery as a potential mode of delivery, especially for triplet gestations."

American College of Obstetricians and Gynecologists. 2004. "Multiple Gestation: Complicated Twin, Triplet, and High-Order Multifetal Pregnancy." *ACOG Practice Bulletin,* no. 56.

Page 215: "The birth essay has, by far, proven to be the single most useful tool that I have in rendering emotional care to pregnant women."

Helgeson, Michele. 2008. The Midwife Archives Web site. www.gentlebirth.org/archives/brthplns.html#Emotional. Personal communication, May 22, 2008.

## Chapter 12

Page 226: Up to 85 percent of all new mothers in the U.S. experience postpartum "blues" during the first ten days or so after birth.

Lee, Kathryn, et al. April–June 2007. "Patterns of Sleep Disruption and Depressive Symptoms in New Mothers." *Journal of Perinatal & Neonatal Nursing,* vol. 21, no. 2, pp. 123–129.

Page 226: According to research explored in the book . . .

Attarian, H.P. 2006. *Sleep Disorders in Women: A Guide to Practical Management (Current Clinical Neurology),* pp. 185–196. Totowa, New Jersey: Humana Press Inc.

Page 227: A study published in 2007 in the *Journal of Perinatal & Neonatal Nursing* . . .

Kennedy, Holly Powell, and Kathryn A. Lee, et al. 2007. "Negotiating Sleep: A Qualitative Study of New Mothers." *Journal of Perinatal & Neonatal Nursing,* vol. 21, no. 2, pp. 114–122.

Page 227: For more on the stages of becoming a mother, see: Mercer, R.T. 2004. "Becoming a Mother versus Maternal Role Attainment." *Journal of Nursing Scholarship,* 36: 226–232.

Page 230: Cockrell, S., C. O'Neill, J. Stone. 2007. *Babyproofing Your Marriage.* New York: HarperCollins.

Page 230: Gottman, J.M., and J.S. Gottman. 2007. *And Baby Makes Three.* New York: Crown.

Page 230: Perel, E. 2006. *Mating in Captivity.* New York: HarperCollins.

Page 230: A study published in 2000 in the *Journal of Family Psychology* . . .

Shapiro, A.F., J.M. Gottman, et al. 2000. "The Baby and the Marriage: Identifying Factors That Buffer Against Decline in Marital Satisfaction After the First Baby Arrives." *Journal of Family Psychology,* vol. 14(1), pp. 59–70.

# ACKNOWLEDGMENTS

*Ananda*

I'd like to sincerely thank the following people for their role in creating this book.

The birth stories that appear in this book are drawn from families whom we know personally, as well as others who responded to our call for input. All their names and identifying details have been changed. My colleagues have also shared numerous birthing techniques with me throughout my career. Thank you to these families, health-care providers, and sister doulas, for allowing me to learn much of what I know from you, so that it can benefit my future clients and the readers of this book.

To Rachel Zimmerman, thank you. As women frequently tell their doulas: I couldn't have done it without you.

Thank you to those who went above and beyond the editorial call of duty: Eve Alpern; William Camann, MD; and Amanda Sawires Yager, HBCE, CCE, CD.

For many hours of editorial help, reviewing for medical accuracy, interviews, education, and moral support, thank you to: ALACE; Stuart Andrews; Martine Bernard; the Birth Sisters program and the Breastfeeding Center at Boston

Medical Center; Marnie Cabezas Skorupa, CPM; Susan Cassel, CNM; the Center for Breastfeeding/Healthy Children 2000 Project; Gina Forbes, CD; Atul Gawande, MD; Marjorie Greenfield, MD; Thérèse Hak-Kuhn, CBA, CBE; Judith Elaine Halek, CCE; Barbara Harper, RN; Harriette Hartigan; Michael Hayes; Madeline Hopkins; Ruti Karni Horowitz; the Kripalu School of Massage; DeeDee Lafayette, MS; Joe Lasell; Alyson Lawson, RN; Gloria Lemay; Beverly Leung; Catherine MacLellan; Corinne McKamey; *Mothering* magazine; Julie Mottl-Santiago, CNM; Kimberly Packard, CBE, CD; Debra Pascali-Bonaro, CCE, CD; Gretchen Putnam, LMT; Gabriel Quirk; Colleen Rafferty; Philip Rappaport; Beth Rashbaum; Nina Sassoon; Todd Shuster; Rachel Smook; Robin Snyder-Drummond; Ilana Stein, CD; Rachel Sussman; Erin Sweeney, LCMT; Andrew Szanton; Nita Taublib; Seth Teller and the Teller Zimmerman family; Tracy Walton, LMT; Jessica Waters; Debbie Young, CD; Noor Zaidi; and Theresa Zoro. Please forgive me if I have forgotten anyone.

And to my mother, Rochelle Lowe; my sisters, Rivka Lachmann and Shulamit Louria, and their families; Elvin Atkins, my beloved; my wonderful friends (yes, you!); and the doula community in Boston and beyond, thank you for loving and encouraging me while I fulfilled my dream of publishing my first book.

*Rachel*

Many mothers, fathers, partners, loved ones, doulas, doctors, midwives, and nurses graciously granted interviews for this book. They are not all named here, but their openness and time is greatly appreciated. Special thanks to Beth Hardiman, Jane Look, Joyce Kimball, Bill Camann, Elizabeth Davis, Penny Simkin, John Kennell, Jane Fonda, Rachel Abramson, Kim Nolte, Richard Reed, Tammy Paul, Jennifer Fargar, Sharon Davis, Leah Kohlstrom, Kathleen Sullivan, Cathy Moore, Joan Singer, Hilary Berkman, and

Tina Cassidy. Amy Brand and Sally Handy introduced me to the world of doulas when I arrived in Cambridge. Elizabeth Call was in my first birthing class, and we emerged together from cluelessness (for the most part). Ananda Lowe provided inspiration and gentle nudging. Todd Shuster helped make the book happen. The *Wall Street Journal* kindly gave me two months off to work on this project. Thanks to my father, Bob Zimmerman, and stepmother, Betsy Fajans, who know about the ups and downs of writing. And most of all, thanks and love to my husband, Seth Teller, an astute editor and enthusiastic proponent of living the examined life and never giving up.

## ABOUT THE AUTHORS

Ananda Lowe has been a leader in the doula movement since 1995. For seven years, she served as assistant director of the Association of Labor Assistants and Childbirth Educators, which conducts the oldest national birth doula training program. She has worked with prominent doulas and medical professionals as well as hundreds of mothers across North America. Ms. Lowe has been interviewed by major publications including *American Baby, Child, NurseWeek, Parenting, Parents,* and *Shape's Fit Pregnancy.* She lives in the Boston area.

Rachel Zimmerman has worked as a journalist for more than two decades. She spent ten years at the *Wall Street Journal,* mostly covering health and medicine, and has written for a range of other publications, including the *New York Times, Slate,* and the *Seattle Post-Intelligencer.* The recipient of numerous awards for her work, Ms. Zimmerman has reported from Africa, China, Vietnam, Cuba, Europe, and across the United States. In 2008, she was selected as a Knight Science Journalism Fellow at the Massachusetts Institute of Technology. She lives in Cambridge, Massachusetts, with her husband and two daughters, each of whom was born with the help of a doula.

# INDEX

Printed in the United States
by Baker & Taylor Publisher Services